Function Preservation in Laryngeal Cancer

Editor

BABAK SADOUGHI

OTOLARYNGOLOGIC CLINICS OF NORTH AMERICA

www.oto.theclinics.com

August 2015 • Volume 48 • Number 4

ELSEVIER

1600 John F. Kennedy Boulevard • Suite 1800 • Philadelphia, Pennsylvania, 19103-2899

http://www.oto.theclinics.com

OTOLARYNGOLOGIC CLINICS OF NORTH AMERICA Volume 48, Number 4
August 2015 ISSN 0030-6665, ISBN-13: 978-0-323-38900-6

Editor: Joanne Husovski
Developmental Editor: Susan Showalter

Otolaryngologic Clinics of North America (ISSN 0030-6665) is published bimonthly by Elsevier, Inc., 360 Park Avenue South, New York, NY 10010-1710. Months of issue are February, April, June, August, October, and December. Business and Editorial Offices: 1600 John F. Kennedy Blvd., Suite 1800, Philadelphia, PA 19103-2899. Customer Service Office: 6277 Sea Harbor Drive, Orlando, FL 32887-4800. Periodicals postage paid at New York, NY and additional mailing offices. Subscription prices is $365.00 per year (US individuals), $692.00 per year (US institutions), $175.00 per year (US student/resident), $485.00 per year (Canadian individuals), $876.00 per year (Canadian institutions), $540.00 per year (international individuals), $876.00 per year (international institutions), $270.00 per year (international & Canadian student/resident). Foreign air speed delivery is included in all *Clinics'* subscription prices. All prices are subject to change without notice. **POSTMASTER:** Send address changes to *Otolaryngologic Clinics of North America,* Elsevier Health Sciences Division, Subscription Customer Service, 3251 Riverport Lane, Maryland Heights, MO 63043. **Telephone: 1-800-654-2452 (U.S. and Canada); 314-447-8871 (outside U.S. and Canada). Fax: 314-447-8029. E-mail: journalscustomerservice-usa@elsevier.com (for print support); journalsonlinesupport-usa@elsevier.com (for online support).**

Reprints. For copies of 100 or more of articles in this publication, please contact the Commercial Reprints Department, Elsevier Inc., 360 Park Avenue South, New York, NY 10010-1710. Tel.: 212-633-3874; Fax: 212-633-3820; E-mail: reprints@elsevier.com.

Otolaryngologic Clinics of North America is also published in Spanish by McGraw-Hill Interamericana Editores S.A., P.O. Box 5-237, 06500 Mexico D.F., Mexico.

Otolaryngologic Clinics of North America is covered in *MEDLINE/PubMed (Index Medicus), Current Contents/Clinical Medicine, Excerpta Medica, BIOSIS, Science Citation Index,* and *ISI/BIOMED.*

PROGRAM OBJECTIVE

The goal of the *Otolaryngologic Clinics of North America* is to provide information on the latest trends in patient management, the newest advances; and provide a sound basis for choosing treatment options in the field of otolaryngology.

LEARNING OBJECTIVES

Upon completion of this activity, participants will be able to:
1. Review methods of preserving voice in the treatment of laryngeal cancer.
2. Discuss quality of life following surgical management of laryngeal cancer.
3. Recognize innovations in contemporary surgical treatments of glottic cancer, including Transoral and Transcervical methods.

ACCREDITATION

The Elsevier Office of Continuing Medical Education (EOCME) is accredited by the Accreditation Council for Continuing Medical Education (ACCME) to provide continuing medical education for physicians.

The EOCME designates this enduring material for a maximum of 15 *AMA PRA Category 1 Credit*(s)™. Physicians should claim only the credit commensurate with the extent of their participation in the activity.

All other health care professionals requesting continuing education credit for this enduring material will be issued a certificate of participation.

DISCLOSURE OF CONFLICTS OF INTEREST

The EOCME assesses conflict of interest with its instructors, faculty, planners, and other individuals who are in a position to control the content of CME activities. All relevant conflicts of interest that are identified are thoroughly vetted by EOCME for fair balance, scientific objectivity, and patient care recommendations. EOCME is committed to providing its learners with CME activities that promote improvements or quality in healthcare and not a specific proprietary business or a commercial interest.

The planning committee, staff, authors and editors listed below have identified no financial relationships or relationships to products or devices they or their spouse/life partner have with commercial interest related to the content of this CME activity:
Andrew Blitzer, MD, DDS; Daniel F. Brasnu, MD; Michelle Mizhi Chen, MD; Mark S. Courey, MD; Seth H. Dailey, MD; Anjali Fortna; Mauricio Gamez, MD; Louis B. Harrison, MD; Dana M. Hartl, MD, PhD; Kristen Helm; F. Christopher Holsinger, MD, FACS; Kenneth Hu, MD; Adrianne Brigido; Ollivier Laccourreye, MD; Samia Laoufi, MD; Niv Mor, MD; Moustafa Mourad, MD; Vyas M. N. Prasad, MSc, FRCS (ORL-HNS); Santha Priya; Marc Remacle, PhD, MD; Babak Sadoughi, MD; Susan Showalter; Catherine F. Sinclair, MD; Melin Tan, MD; Christopher G. Tang, MD; Kathleen M. Tibbetts, MD; Craig R. Villari, MD; Chad W. Whited, MD.

The planning committee, staff, authors and editors listed below have identified financial relationships or relationships to products or devices they or their spouse/life partner have with commercial interest related to the content of this CME activity:
Steven M. Zeitels, MD, FACS has stock ownership in Endocraft LLC, and receives research support from Voice Health Institute; The V Foundation for Cancer Research; the Eugene B. Casey Foundation; and the National Philanthropic Trust, and has stock ownership in Endocraft LLC.

UNAPPROVED/OFF-LABEL USE DISCLOSURE

The EOCME requires CME faculty to disclose to the participants:
1. When products or procedures being discussed are off-label, unlabelled, experimental, and/or investigational (not US Food and Drug Administration [FDA] approved); and
2. Any limitations on the information presented, such as data that are preliminary or that represent ongoing research, interim analyses, and/or unsupported opinions. Faculty may discuss information about pharmaceutical agents that is outside of FDA-approved labelling. This information is intended solely for CME and is not intended to promote off-label use of these medications. If you have any questions, contact the medical affairs department of the manufacturer for the most recent prescribing information.

TO ENROLL

To enroll in the *Otolaryngologic Clinics of North America* Continuing Medical Education program, call customer service at 1-800-654-2452 or sign up online at http://www.theclinics.com/home/cme. The CME program is available to subscribers for an additional annual fee of USD 260.

METHOD OF PARTICIPATION

In order to claim credit, participants must complete the following:
1. Complete enrolment as indicated above.
2. Read the activity.
3. Complete the CME Test and Evaluation. Participants must achieve a score of 70% on the test. All CME Tests and Evaluations must be completed online.

CME INQUIRIES/SPECIAL NEEDS

For all CME inquiries or special needs, please contact elsevierCME@elsevier.com.

Contributors

EDITOR

BABAK SADOUGHI, MD
Assistant Professor of Otolaryngology, Department of Otolaryngology–Head and Neck Surgery, The Sean Parker Institute for the Voice, Weill Cornell Medical College, New York Presbyterian Hospital, New York, New York

AUTHORS

ANDREW BLITZER, MD, DDS
Department of Otolaryngology–Head and Neck Surgery, Mount Sinai Roosevelt Hospital; New York Center for Voice and Swallowing Disorders, Head and Neck Surgical Group, New York, New York

DANIEL F. BRASNU, MD
Chief, Otolaryngology–Head and Neck Surgery; Chief, University Hospital Cancer Pole, Paris Descartes University and Sorbonne Paris III University, Hôpital Européen Georges Pompidou, Paris, France

MICHELLE MIZHI CHEN, MD
Division of Head and Neck Surgery, Department of Otolaryngology–Head and Neck Surgery, Stanford University, Palo Alto, California

MARK S. COUREY, MD
Professor, Department of Otolaryngology–Head and Neck Surgery; Director, Division of Laryngology, University of California - San Francisco, San Francisco, California

SETH H. DAILEY, MD
Associate Professor, Chief, Section of Laryngology and Voice Surgery, Otolaryngology–Head and Neck Surgery, University of Wisconsin at Madison, Madison, Wisconsin

MAURICIO GAMEZ, MD
Department of Radiation Oncology, Mayo Clinic Hospital, Mayo Clinic Arizona, Phoenix, Arizona

LOUIS B. HARRISON, MD
Department of Radiation Oncology, Moffitt Cancer Center, Tampa, Florida

DANA M. HARTL, MD, PhD
Chief, Service Rhône, Department of Head and Neck Oncology, Institut de Cancérologie Gustave Roussy, Villejuif, France

F. CHRISTOPHER HOLSINGER, MD, FACS
Director, Head and Neck Oncology Program; Chief, Division of Head and Neck Surgery; Professor, Department of Otolaryngology–Head and Neck Surgery, Stanford University, Palo Alto, California

KENNETH HU, MD
Department of Radiation Oncology, NYU-Langone Medical Center, New York,
New York

OLLIVIER LACCOURREYE, MD
Department of Otorhinolaryngology–Head and Neck Surgery, University Paris
Descartes Sorbonne Paris Cité, Hôpital Européen Georges Pompidou, Assistance
Publique – Hôpitaux de Paris, Paris, France

SAMIA LAOUFI, MD
Department of Head and Neck Oncology, Institut de Cancérologie Gustave Roussy,
Villejuif, France

NIV MOR, MD
Department of Otolaryngology–Head and Neck Surgery, Mount Sinai Roosevelt Hospital;
New York Center for Voice and Swallowing Disorders, Head and Neck Surgical Group,
New York, New York

MOUSTAFA MOURAD, MD
Resident, Department of Otolaryngology, New York Eye and Ear Infirmary, Mount Sinai
Health System, New York, New York

VYAS M.N. PRASAD, MSc, FRCS (ORL-HNS)
Department of Otolaryngology–Head and Neck Surgery, University Hospital of Louvain at
Mont-Godinne, Yvoir, Belgium; Ng Teng Fong Hospital, Singapore; Alexandra Hospital,
Singapore

MARC REMACLE, PhD, MD
Department of Otolaryngology–Head and Neck Surgery, University Hospital of Louvain at
Mont-Godinne, Yvoir, Belgium

BABAK SADOUGHI, MD
Assistant Professor of Otolaryngology, Department of Otolaryngology–Head and Neck
Surgery, The Sean Parker Institute for the Voice, Weill Cornell Medical College, New York
Presbyterian Hospital, New York, New York

CATHERINE F. SINCLAIR, MD
Assistant Professor, Department of Otolaryngology, Mount Sinai Icahn School of
Medicine, New York, New York

MELIN TAN, MD
Assistant Professor, Department of Otorhinolaryngology–Head and Neck Surgery,
Montefiore Medical Center, Albert Einstein College of Medicine, Bronx, New York

CHRISTOPHER G. TANG, MD
New York Center for Voice and Swallowing Disorders, New York, New York

KATHLEEN M. TIBBETTS, MD
Resident Physician, Department of Otorhinolaryngology–Head and Neck Surgery,
Montefiore Medical Center, Albert Einstein College of Medicine, Bronx, New York

CRAIG R. VILLARI, MD
Assistant Professor, Department of Otolaryngology–Head and Neck Surgery, Emory
University, Atlanta, Georgia

CHAD W. WHITED, MD
Laryngology Fellow, Clinical Instructor, Otolaryngology–Head and Neck Surgery, University of Wisconsin at Madison, Madison, Wisconsin

STEVEN M. ZEITELS, MD, FACS
Eugene B. Casey Professor of Laryngeal Surgery, Harvard Medical School; Director, Division of Laryngeal Surgery, Massachusetts General Hospital, Boston, Massachusetts

Contents

Laryngeal barriers to tumor spread are a product of laryngeal development, anatomic barriers, and enzymatic activity. Supraglottic and glottic/subglottic development is distinct and partially explains the metastatic behavior of laryngeal carcinoma. Dense connective tissues and elastic fibers provide anatomic barriers within the larynx. Laryngeal cartilage contains dense cartilage, enzyme inhibitors, and an intact perichondrium making it relatively resistant to tumor invasion; however, focal areas of vulnerability are created by ossified cartilage and natural interruptions in the perichondrium. Local inflammation and the enzymatic interplay between tumor and host are important factors in the spread of laryngeal tumor.

The evaluation of the dysphonic patient begins with a complete understanding of the laryngeal anatomy and physiology of voice production. A thorough history must be taken regarding the dysphonia qualities, alarming symptoms, and confounding factors. The complete head and neck examination culminates in a detailed visualization of the vocal folds using image-capturing laryngoscopy as well as stroboscopy or high-speed digital imaging to fully evaluate the viscoelastic properties of the vocal fold cover-body structure and function. Finally, the evaluation leads to the biopsy of any concerning lesions either under magnification in the operating room or topical anesthesia in the office.

Laryngeal cancer accounts for approximately 2.4% of new malignancies worldwide each year. Early identification of laryngeal neoplasms results in improved prognosis and functional outcomes. Imaging plays an integral role in the diagnosis, staging, and long-term follow-up of laryngeal cancer. This article highlights advanced laryngeal imaging techniques and their application to early glottic neoplasms.

Preserving Voice in Early Laryngeal Cancer

Mauricio Gamez, Kenneth Hu, and Louis B. Harrison

Laryngeal function after oncologic treatment is a key aspect and focus of interest in the contemporary management of head and neck cancers. Although historically the treatment of most locally advanced laryngeal cancers has been total laryngectomy, recent innovations in radiation therapy and combined chemotherapy and radiation therapy have shown that organ and function preservation can be achieved with good oncologic outcomes. Technical improvements, along with better understanding of tumor biology and dose tolerance of critical organs involved in speech and swallowing function, have paved the way for better outcomes. This article reviews in comprehensive detail the recent data of laryngeal function after radiotherapy.

Craig R. Villari and Mark S. Courey

Radiation-induced dysphonia can develop after radiation for primary laryngeal cancer or when the larynx is in the radiation field for nonlaryngeal malignancy. The effects are dose dependent and lead to variable degrees of dysphonia in both short- and long-term follow-up. Rehabilitation of the irradiated larynx can prove frustrating but can be facilitated through behavioral, pharmacologic, or surgical interventions.

Dana M. Hartl and Daniel F. Brasnu

For early-stage T1-T2 glottic squamous cell carcinoma, transoral laser microsurgery (TLM) is the main surgical modality, with rates of local control and laryngeal preservation ranging from 85% to 100% and low morbidity. For extensive lesions, open conservation laryngeal surgery may enable wider resections than TLM but at costs of longer hospital stay and higher postoperative morbidity. Surgery provides results that are comparable to nonsurgical treatment options while reserving radiation therapy for recurrences or second primary cancers, particularly in younger patients. In the future, transoral robot-assisted surgery may enable more extensive transoral resections than laser alone, decreasing further the indications for open surgery.

Dana M. Hartl, Samia Laoufi, and Daniel F. Brasnu

Transoral laser microsurgery (TLM) is the mainstay in the treatment of early (TisT1T2) glottic cancer. Current knowledge concerning voice quality and voice-related quality of life in patients treated using TLM is based on small cohort studies using various instruments to evaluate these functional results. The bulk of the literature indicates that subjective and objective

Preserving and Restoring Function in Advanced Laryngeal Cancer

OTOLARYNGOLOGIC CLINICS
OF NORTH AMERICA

RELATED INTEREST

Surgical Oncology Clinics of North America
July 2015 (Vol. 24, Issue 3)
Head and Neck Cancer
John A. Ridge, *Editor*

THE CLINICS ARE AVAILABLE ONLINE!
Access your subscription at:
www.theclinics.com

Preface

Function Preservation in Laryngeal Cancer

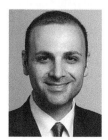

Babak Sadoughi, MD
Editor

Treating laryngeal cancer entails a rare set of challenges. The larynx is not only complex in structure and function, but also essential to some of the most fundamental attributes defining us as human beings. In addition, laryngeal malignancy follows peculiar patterns of progression, making it a somewhat atypical entity within the realm of head and neck oncology, and rendering its global comprehension singularly difficult.

Accordingly, the management of laryngeal cancer has had a history torn between inflexible orthodoxy and hasty modernism. In the early days, when total laryngectomy—later supplemented by adjuvant radiation therapy—was the only weapon at hand, curing laryngeal cancer was simply an exercise in radicality, aimed at prolonging life at all costs without much consideration for the functional consequences of treatment itself. The ingenious developments of open partial laryngectomy and transoral laser microsurgery were soon able to offer alternative options for surgical management with no compromise on oncologic outcomes. However, a dramatic change in paradigm was initiated after the publication of the seminal chemoradiation reports and the advent of nonsurgical organ-preservation protocols, felt to be the conveyors of the long-awaited age of reason for the treatment of laryngeal cancer. Unfortunately, assertive implementation of definitive chemoradiation, with particular enthusiasm in this country, did not prove it to be the panacea, as survival rates have remained largely unchanged for the past thirty years, while the community realized that preserving the gross structure of the larynx was not sufficient to guarantee proper function.

Concurrently, quality-of-life expectations rose, and morbidity and function metrics of outcome became just as crucial as the traditional oncologic ones. With survival rates remaining fairly equivalent regardless of the treatment modality employed—provided patient selection is performed according to commonly accepted rules—it is now only logical to begin viewing the management of laryngeal cancer primarily through the prism of function preservation.

Otolaryngol Clin N Am 48 (2015) xv–xvii
http://dx.doi.org/10.1016/j.otc.2015.06.001
0030-6665/15/$ – see front matter © 2015 Published by Elsevier Inc.

oto.theclinics.com

It is precisely the goal of this issue of *Otolaryngologic Clinics of North America* to place the emphasis on function. Rather than expressing peremptory and dismissive positions on individual treatment strategies, or expecting the unpredictable momentum of an erratic pendulum to pave new roads that may ultimately prove treacherous, there is tremendous opportunity in capitalizing on the vast treatment armamentarium, broadened knowledge base, and technology capabilities compiled through decades of experience, trials, and errors, in order to offer each patient a truly tailored approach meeting individual needs and expectations.

This issue tackles the critical goal of function preservation from various angles. First, the most reliable way to minimize the impact of disease or its treatment on laryngeal function remains early diagnosis. The unique anatomic and histologic aspects of tumor progression within the larynx are reviewed, as well as the clinical methods and increasingly sophisticated tools available to detect laryngeal cancer at its earliest stages.

Once the diagnosis of laryngeal cancer is confirmed, the stage of disease will be the main driver of the treatment strategy. The most recent data on the management of early glottic cancer are presented, along with the anticipated functional impact of surgical and nonsurgical modalities. We also review the state-of-the-art approaches to the rehabilitation of dysphonia resulting from those treatment modalities.

In its advanced stages, laryngeal cancer often continues to represent an essentially local hazard with major functional implications, possibly exacerbated by treatment. It is important to realize the potentially dramatic consequences of treatment not only on voice and swallowing functions, but also on overall quality of life, which we discuss and propose to recognize as a critical parameter of treatment selection. While total laryngectomy remains the gold standard of salvage treatment of radiorecurrent disease, we would be remiss to ignore the irreversible nature of its psychosocial effects, particularly in the presence of treatment alternatives that a carefully selected subset of patients may benefit from, whether through time-honored conservation laryngeal surgery procedures, or cutting-edge innovations in technique and treatment philosophy presented in this issue. Finally, crossing the Rubicon and performing a total laryngectomy will often solve some inextricable challenges, particularly pertaining to deglutition, but should not amount to renouncing the focus on voice function and quality-of-life preservation; thus, an overview of the current state of voice restoration after total laryngectomy is offered.

We close this issue of *Otolaryngologic Clinics of North America* with an exciting new "Early Practice" section, developed primarily for physicians in training or in their initial years of practice, in which we discuss some of the most relevant techniques of open partial laryngectomy, with a focus on anatomy through a simplified outline structure complemented with illustrative media material.

The elaboration of this unique collection of topics would not have been feasible without a gathering of world-class authors, who graciously agreed to honor me with their outstanding contributions. I am in debt to all of them, not only for their precious help with this project, but also for all they have done to help me affirm myself as a physician, as they represent a fine selection of esteemed mentors, colleagues, and friends of mine.

It is my hope that this collaborative effort will foster a rational and balanced understanding of where we should stand in our capacity of advocates of the patient with laryngeal cancer. If this issue succeeds merely in convincing a few skeptics, infuriating a handful of dogmatists, and giving hope to some cynics, then, undoubtedly, it will have served its purpose.

Babak Sadoughi, MD
The Sean Parker Institute for the Voice
Department of Otolaryngology–Head & Neck Surgery
Weill Cornell Medical College
1305 York Avenue, 5th Floor
New York, NY 10021, USA

E-mail address:
bas9049@med.cornell.edu

Diagnosing Laryngeal Cancer

Functional Anatomy and Oncologic Barriers of the Larynx

 CrossMark

Niv Mor, MD[a,b,*], Andrew Blitzer, MD, DDS[a,b]

KEYWORDS

- Larynx • Tumor • Barriers • Facilitator • Inflammation

KEY POINTS

- Supraglottic development is distinct from glottic and subglottic development, which partially explains the metastatic behavior of laryngeal carcionoma.
- Dense connective tissues and elastic fibers provide anatomic barriers within the larynx.
- Ossified cartilage and interruptions in the perichondrium create vulnerable points to tumor spread.
- Tumor spread is not purely mechanical.
- Tumor stimulates the host to activate enzymes that break down the body's natural barriers to invasion.

INTRODUCTION

A thorough knowledge of laryngeal anatomy, embryology, and biology can help us understand the barriers and facilitators of tumor spread within the larynx.

LARYNGEAL ANATOMY

Laryngeal Regions

The larynx is dived into 3 regions (supraglottis, glottis, and subglottis). The supraglottis is subdivided into 5 segments (suprahyoid epiglottis, infrahyoid epiglottis, laryngeal surface of the aryepiglottic folds, arytenoids, and false vocal cords). A horizontal plane through the lateral margin of the ventricle marks the inferior extent of the supraglottis. Below this plane marks the beginning of the glottis. The glottis is composed of the true vocal folds and the space between them, which is called the rima glottidis. The true

Disclosures: None.
[a] Department of Otolaryngology – Head and Neck Surgery, Mount Sinai Roosevelt Hospital, 425 59th Street, 10th Floor, New York, NY 10019, USA; [b] New York Center for Voice and Swallowing Disorders, Head and Neck Surgical Group, 425 59th Street, 10th Floor, New York, NY 10019, USA
* Corresponding author.
E-mail address: nivmor73@gmail.com

Otolaryngol Clin N Am 48 (2015) 533–545
http://dx.doi.org/10.1016/j.otc.2015.04.002
0030-6665/15/$ – see front matter © 2015 Elsevier Inc. All rights reserved.

oto.theclinics.com

vocal folds include the epithelium, superficial lamina propria, vocal ligament (intermediate and deep lamina propria), and the vocalis muscle. The glottis extends from the anterior commissure, the junction of the vocal folds and vocal ligaments with the thyroid cartilage, to the vocal process of the arytenoid cartilage. The glottis continues in the caudal direction for a distance of approximately 1 cm. The subglottis begins at the inferior border of the glottis and continues caudally to the inferior border of the cricoid cartilage.[1]

Borders of the Larynx

The superior surfaces of the epiglottis and aryepiglottic folds correspond to the cranial boundary of the larynx. The lingual surfaces of the suprahyoid epiglottis and the hyoepiglottic ligament form the anterosuperior limit of the larynx and form the roof of the preepiglottic space. The anterior border of the larynx is bounded to the thyrohyoid membrane and thyroid cartilage at the level of the supraglottis, the thyroid cartilage at the level of the glottis, and the cricothyroid membrane and cricoid cartilage at the level of the subglottis.[1] The inferior edge of the cricoid cartilage marks the inferior limit of the larynx. The laryngeal surfaces of the aryepiglottic folds and arytenoid cartilages mark the lateral and posterolateral borders of the larynx. The interarytenoid space and the posterior wall of the cricoid ring mark the posterior border of the larynx. The lateral surfaces of the aryepiglottic folds are not part of the larynx. They belong to the pyriform sinus, which is a subdivision of the hypopharynx.[2]

Laryngeal Spaces

The laryngeal aperture is the superior laryngeal inlet and is bounded by the epiglottis anteriorly, the aryepiglottic folds laterally, and the interarytenoid space posteriorly. The larynx openly communicates with the pharynx at the superior and posterosuperior laryngeal aperture. Caudal to the laryngeal aperture is the laryngeal vestibule, which corresponds to the space between the laryngeal aperture and the vestibular folds (false vocal folds). The laryngeal vestibule is bounded anteriorly by the epiglottis and laterally by the aryepiglottic folds. The laryngeal ventricle, also referred to as Morgagni sinus, is the space between the vestibular folds (false vocal folds) superiorly and the true vocal folds inferiorly. At the anterior roof of the ventricle lies a pouchlike structure called the saccule, which functions to lubricate the ipsilateral vocal fold. The lateral most aspect of the ventricle is the embryologic fusion point of the buccopharyngeal and the tracheobronchial primordium, which marks the border between the supraglottis and glottis. The glottic opening is called the rima glottidis. The rima glottidis is divided into the intermembranous space between the true vocal folds and the intercartilaginous space between the vocal processes of the arytenoids. The rima glottidis is the narrowest part of the laryngeal cavity.

Potential Spaces

The preepiglottic space is a potential space immediately in front of the epiglottis and is bound by the hyoepiglottic ligament (superior), the thyrohyoid membrane and the lamina of the thyroid cartilage (anterior), and the thyroepiglottic ligament (inferior). This potential space is composed of adipose tissue and is devoid of lymph nodes. The anterior aspect of the laryngeal saccule extends from the laryngeal ventricle into the preepiglottic space. The preepiglottic space extends slightly beyond the lateral margins of the epiglottis often referred to as horseshoe shaped. Therefore, the term peri-epiglottic space is a slightly more accurate description of this region.[3] The caudal part of the periepiglottic space is subdivided into 1 median region and 2 lateral regions. The median region is immediately anterior to the epiglottis. The 2 lateral subdivisions correspond to the adipose and glandular tissue of the vestibular folds (false vocal folds) and are separated from the potential space of the paraglottic space by the thyroarytenoid muscle and the fibrous extensions of its muscle sheet.

The paraglottic space is a potential space bound by the thyroid cartilage and cricothyroid membrane (lateral), the quadrangular membrane and the conus elasticus (medial), and the pyriform sinus (posterior). Posteroinferiorly the paraglottic space extends to the cricothyroid joint. The paraglottic space, which is made up primarily of adipose tissue, contains the internal branch of the superior laryngeal nerve.[3]

Just under the epithelial cover of the glottis is another potential space referred to as the Reinke space. This potential space corresponds to superficial lamina propria and is made up of a soft gelatinlike substance composed primarily of a loose fibrous and elastic matrix.

Laryngeal Structures

Cartilage and membranes

The laryngeal framework is composed of hyaline and elastic cartilage. It has 3 unpaired cartilages (epiglottis, thyroid, and cricoid cartilage) and 3 paired cartilages (arytenoid, corniculate, and cuneiform cartilage). Only epiglottis is composed of elastic cartilage, and the remaining cartilaginous structures are made up of hyaline cartilage. The larynx also has 6 fibrous membranes (hyoepiglottic ligament, thyroepiglottic ligament, thyrohyoid membrane, quadrangular membrane, conus elasticus, and cricothyroid membrane). With the exception of the thyroepiglottic ligament, the laryngeal cartilages and fibrous membranes form strong natural barriers to the spread of tumor. The larynx is devoid of a true bony structure. Although the hyoid bone functions as a point of stability to the larynx, it is not a laryngeal structure.

Muscles

The muscles of the larynx are separated into intrinsic and extrinsic laryngeal muscles. The intrinsic laryngeal muscles are responsible for varying the glottic opening, protecting the airway, and producing voice. The extrinsic laryngeal muscles support the position of the larynx by elevating or depressing the larynx and are used primarily in swallowing.

The intrinsic laryngeal muscles include the lateral cricoarytenoid and interarytenoid muscles, which adduct the vocal folds, the cricothyroid and thyroarytenoid muscles, which add tension to the vocal folds, and the posterior cricoarytenoid, which abducts the vocal folds. The posterior cricoarytenoid muscle is traditionally represented as one muscle; however, Sanders and colleagues[4] showed the posterior cricoarytenoid muscle is composed of 3 muscle components (vertical, oblique, and horizontal component). They speculated that the vertical and oblique components are responsible for vocal fold abduction and the horizontal component is responsible for arytenoid stabilization during phonation.

The muscles of the supraglottis are formed from extensions of the intrinsic laryngeal muscles. The oblique arytenoid muscles have their origin at the posterior aspect of the arytenoid muscular process and cross midline to insert at the apex of the contralateral arytenoid cartilage. Some of the fibers then continue as the aryepiglottic muscle. The aryepiglottic muscles function primarily in narrowing the laryngeal vestibule. Similarly, some muscle fibers from the thyroarytenoid muscle extend into the lateral aspect of the aryepiglottic fold and epiglottis. These fibers are referred to as the thyroepiglottic muscles and function to widen the laryngeal vestibule.

The extrinsic laryngeal muscles are divided into the suprahyoid muscles that elevate the larynx (digastric, stylohyoid, mylohyoid, geniohyoid, and hyoglossus muscles) and the infrahyoid muscles that depress the larynx (thyrohyoid, sternothyroid, omohyoid, and sternohyoid muscles).

Mucosa and submucosal layers

The epithelium of the supraglottis is composed of respiratory pseudostratified columnar epithelium and has an abundance of mucous glands and lymphatic vessels. The only exception is at the edges of the aryepiglottic folds and at the lateral borders of the epiglottis, which are composed of stratified squamous epithelium.

The vocal folds are often wrongfully referred to as cords. This term came from the French anatomist, Antoine Ferrein, who named them *cordes vocales* when he thought the glottis generated sound by vibrating like strings of a violin. We now know that sound is generated by a mucosal wave formed by the glottic epithelium suspended over a vocal ligament. The glottis is, therefore, more accurately referred to as vocal folds. The epithelium is composed of stratified squamous epithelium. Deep to the epithelium lays the lamina propria, which is devoid of lymphatic vessels and is divided into superficial, intermediate, and deep layers. The superficial lamina propria is made up of a soft gelatinlike substance that is composed primarily of a loose fibrous and elastic matrix. The intermediate and deep layers of the lamina propria make up the vocal ligament. The intermediate lamina propria adds elastic mechanical integrity to the vocal fold and is made up primarily of elastic fibers. The deep lamina propria is made up primarily of collagenous fibers and adds durability to the ligament.[5] The vocal ligament forms the superior border of the conus elasticus, which interlocks with the vocalis muscle.

At the anterior roof of the ventricle lies a pouchlike structure called the saccule. The saccule is made of both mucous and serous glands. In children the saccule may contain laryngeal lymphoid tissue, but in adults the presence of a lymphoid tissue in the saccule is pathologic and may indicate the presence of carcinoma. The function of the saccule is mainly to lubricate the ipsilateral vocal fold during speech and deglutition. The saccule may also contribute to increasing voice resonance.[6]

The subglottis is lined by respiratory pseudostratified columnar epithelium. The subglottis is the only area of the larynx that is rigid because of the formation of a complete cartilaginous ring of the cricoid cartilage.

BARRIERS AND PATHWAYS TO TUMOR SPREAD
Embryologic Barriers

Understanding laryngeal embryology can help explain the behavior of tumor spread within the larynx. The development of the supraglottis and glottis is distinct with each carrying an independent blood supply and lymphatic channel. The differentiation between the supraglottis and glottis was first described by Hajek, in 1932, when he observed that laryngeal edema was localized within compartments.[7,8] In 1956 Pressman and colleagues[9] elaborated on this observation by injecting dye into the larynx and found the junction of the vocal and vestibular folds to mark the border between the supraglottis and the glottis.[8] At the infraglottis the dye would flow from the vocal fold to the end of the cricoid and stop at the midline. These boundaries correspond to the embryologic fusion points and help explain the behavior of tumor spread within the larynx.

The supraglottis is derived from the buccopharyngeal primordium, and its lymphatics flow laterally into the deep cervical lymph nodes of level II and level III bilaterally before reaching inferiorly to the lateral lymph nodes of level IV.[10] The supraglottis is rich in lymphatic channels, which explains the propensity for supraglottic cancers to present with nodal metastasis. In addition, the supraglottis is formed from a single midline structure; its lymphatic drainage is, therefore, bilateral.[11] The buccopharyngeal primordium of the supraglottis is derived from the third and fourth brachial arches, and its blood supply comes from the superior laryngeal artery.

In contrast to the supraglottis, the glottis and subglottis are derived from 2 laterally based furrows of the tracheobronchial primordium that fuse at the midline with a median-based furrow. Its lymphatics, therefore, drain unilaterally.[10,11] Additionally, the lymphatics to the glottis are sparse, which explains why glottic lesions rarely present with positive metastatic lymph nodes. The lymphatics of the glottis are focused centrally to the prelaryngeal and pretracheal nodes of level VI. The tracheobronchial primordium of the glottis and subglottis is derived from the sixth brachial arch, and its blood supply comes from the inferior laryngeal arteries.

These boundaries are distinct embryologic boundaries and are often respected by lymphatic metastases. Nevertheless, these embryologic boundaries alone are poor barriers to local tumor spread.

Anatomic Barriers and Facilitators to Tumor Spread

In addition to the developmental boundaries, the larynx has clear anatomic barriers to the spread of malignancy. Within the larynx, tumor spread is bounded by the ligaments, connective tissue membranes, and laryngeal cartilages and facilitated by soft tissue spaces and muscle.

Fibrous barriers to tumor spread

Tucker and Smith[12] found elastic and dense connective tissues to be relatively resistant to tumor invasion. This finding explains why ligaments composed of ground substance, elastic fibers, and dense collagen are strong anatomic barriers to laryngeal tumors. Particularly effective barriers include the submucosal elastic layer, conus elasticus, quadrangular membrane, ventricular connective tissue, hyoepiglottic ligament, and glossoepiglottic ligament. Similarly, the vocal ligament tendon, also known as Broyles ligament, is a strong barrier to tumor invasion. However, as is discussed later in this article, the perichondrium at the anterior commissure is naturally interrupted by the muscular attachments to the thyroid cartilage at the vocal ligament tendon creating a focal area of vulnerability to tumor spread.

Beitler and colleagues[13] described barriers to ventricular invasion from tumors of the paraglottic space. The barrier is formed by 2 subepithelial periventricular membranes referred to as the central periventricular membrane and the peripheral periventricular membrane. The central periventricular membrane is composed of elastic fibers. As is mentioned later, elastic fibers are naturally stable and serve as a relatively good barrier to invasion. The peripheral periventricular membrane, which is contiguous with the conus elasticus and quadrangular membranes, is composed of fibroelastic fibers. The quadrangular membrane is made up of closely woven undulating collagen and elastic fibers. Along with the conus elasticus, the quadrangular membrane provides a strong oncologic separation between the supraglottic and glottic and protects the glottis from carcinoma that is approaching from the vestibule.[14] By contrast, the thyroepiglottic ligament is a relatively poor barrier to tumor spread with carcinoma of the vestibule often eroding upward through the thyroepiglottic ligament. The relative weakness of the thyroepiglottic ligament has to do with it microscopic composition. The thyroepiglottic ligament is made up of sagittally oriented collagen fiber bundles separated by adipose tissue, and tumor spread is facilitated in between these collagen fiber bundles. When compared with the dense interlaced fibrous mass of the hyoepiglottic ligament, the thyroepiglottic ligament seems weak.[3]

The elastic fibers found in arteries make them a relatively resistant structure to tumor invasion. Malignant invasion is partially a result of the tumor's ability to stimulate host-activated collagenase. However, tumor rarely elicits elastase activation. In addition, elastic fibers have a slow turnover rate making them less susceptible to exposures of damage and repair.[8]

The laryngeal epithelium is also relatively resistant to tumor invasion, with laryngeal tumor often demonstrating subepithelial expansion before infiltration.[8]

In addition, the dense fibrous layer encasing the surrounding viscera, like the thyroid gland, provides an additional barrier to tumor infiltration.[8]

Cartilaginous barriers to tumor spread

Laryngeal cartilages are relatively resistant to tumor invasion often demonstrating extensive tumor spread along and around the laryngeal cartilage surfaces before invasion[8] (**Fig. 1**).

Tumors require a rich source of nutrition and oxygen in order to proliferate, and the ability of cartilage to be relatively tumor resistant has partially to do with its lack of an intrinsic blood supply.[15] Laryngeal cartilage is also composed of a matrix that acts as a physical barrier. In addition, cartilage contains enzyme inhibitors that block collagenase, protease, and tumor angiogenesis factor protecting it from degeneration and invasion.[16–21] Besides the intrinsic properties of cartilage to resist tumor invasion, the perichondrium is a strong barrier to tumor spread.

Nevertheless, laryngeal perichondrium has focal areas that are vulnerable to tumor invasion. Collagen bundles pass through the perichondrium at muscular attachment points creating a natural interruption in the perichondrium. Invasion occurs preferentially in these areas. Tumor is often seen separating these collagen bundles allowing direct access to the cartilage.[22] Broyles noted tumor invasion at the insertion point of the vocal ligament tendon to the thyroid cartilage which explained the propensity for tumor to invade at the anterior commissure.[22–24]

The normal adult larynx has a variable ossification pattern that begins around the third decade of life. However, laryngeal ossification can also result from neoplastic

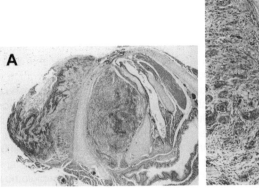
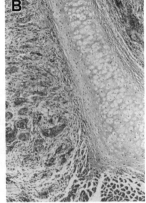

Fig. 1. (*A*) Micrograph of laryngeal tumor showing resistance of cartilage to tumor invasion (hematoxylin-eosin, original magnification ×26). (*B*) High-power magnification of (*A*) (hematoxylin-eosin, original magnification ×130). (*Adapted from* Blitzer A. Regional behavioral variations of epidermoid carcinoma of the head and neck: a study in an animal model. Laryngoscope 1982;92(11):1219–38; with permission.)

disease. Computerized tomography has been shown to be a relatively sensitive modality to identify neoplastic cartilage ossification and to differentiate it from healthy laryngeal cartilage.[25,26] Pathologic cartilage sclerosis begins with tumor-initiated inflammation. Osteoblastic ossification of laryngeal cartilage is followed by the release of prostaglandins and interleukin 1 from the tumor. The tumor-initiated inflammatory process then activates osteoclasts to erode the newly formed bone within the cartilaginous framework. Osteoclasts accumulated at the surface of ossified cartilage and destroyed it ahead of the advancing edge of the tumor[27] (**Fig. 2**). Cartilage adjacent to the tumor is also affected by the nearby inflammation, and the ossification process continues even in the absence of direct contact with the tumor. Ossified cartilage also lacks the enzymatic inhibitors to tumor invasion like tumor angiogenesis factor inhibitor and collagenase inhibitor found in healthy cartilage, increasing its vulnerability to invasion.[15,26,28]

Observational studies have shown that in the early stages, laryngeal framework invasion occurs primarily at the lower third of the thyroid cartilage and the upper edge of the cricoid ring which corresponds to the muscular attachment points. As stated earlier, susceptibility to invasion at these points has to do with the natural deficiency in the perichondrium at areas of muscular attachment. In addition, the stress at these locations leads to focal areas of ossification creating additional vulnerability of cartilage to invasion. Yeager and Archer[22] observed that sites of attachment of the strongest membranes like the vocal ligament tendon and the cricothyroid membrane corresponded to the most frequent sites of invasion.

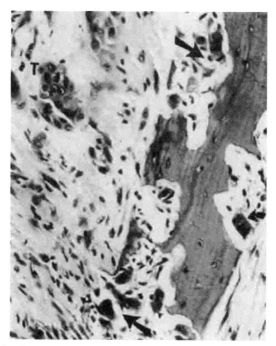

Fig. 2. Micrograph of a multinucleate osteoclasts eroding ossified thyroid cartilage. Arrow shows osteoclasts at the leading edge of tumor invasion (Hematoxylin-eosin, original magnification ×240). T, tumor. (*From* Pittam MR, Carter RL. Framework invasion by laryngeal carcinomas. Head Neck Surg 1982;4(3):200–8; with permission.)

An additional area within the cartilaginous larynx that is vulnerable to tumor invasion is through the natural cribriform conformation of the epiglottis. Carcinoma of or near the epiglottis has easy access to the periepiglottic space through these fenestrations[29] (**Fig. 3**).

Soft tissue space

Although cancer spread is not purely a mechanical phenomenon, tumor spread is facilitated through open areas of loose connective tissue; areas composed of loose collagen and reticulin fibers are easily invaded by tumors.[8]

Venous structures

Unlike arteries, veins lack the protective barriers of elastic fibers. They are easily compressible, and adjacent bulky tumors often cause narrowing of the lumen leading to intimal damage, proliferation, and adhesions between opposing vessel walls. A local phlebitis at this area helps facilitate tumor infiltration.[8]

Muscle

Muscle is a relatively poor barrier to tumor invasion. Once the tumor has crossed the basement membrane, it can readily spread between muscle fibers, displacing the

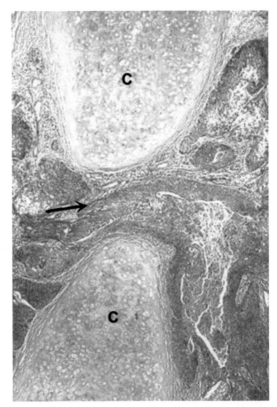

Fig. 3. Micrograph of supraglottic tumor invading through a natural fenestration of the epiglottic cartilage (c) (*arrow* indicates fenestration) (Hematoxylin-eosin). (*From* Barnes L. Diseases of the larynx, hypopharynx, and trachea. In: Barnes L, editor. Surgical pathology of the head and neck. New York: Informa Healthcare; 2009. p. 109–200; with permission.)

sarcolemma and initiating a local inflammatory response. The inflammation incites degenerative changes to nearby muscle fibers even in the absence of tumor invasion. Similar to the process seen in neoplastic cartilage ossification, the nearby muscle fibers do not need to contact the tumor to begin the degenerative process. Degenerated muscle fibers take on a gelatinous amorphous form and passively allow tumors to spread without inhibition.[8]

Anterior commissure

The anterior commissure is a known area of weakness to tumor invasion, which has to do with focal interruptions in the perichondrium and ineffective barriers to tumor invasion inferior to Broyles ligament.

Rucci and colleagues[30,31] described the embryology of the anterior commissure and showed Broyles ligament to be composed of a dense connective tissue system derived from an embryologic collection of cells rich in elastic fibers known as the medial process. Broyles ligament is contiguous with the intermediate lamina of the thyroid cartilage and ends just above the glottic plane. Beyond this point, Broyles ligament is replaced by a relatively thin layer of dense connective tissue and a thinner intermediate lamina making the cartilaginous framework inferior to Broyles ligament vulnerable to tumor invasions.[24,30–32] Therefore, the vulnerability to tumor invasion at the thyroid cartilage starts at the anterior commissure and extends caudally. Rarely does tumor invade cranial to the glottic plane where it would need to invade the dense fibers of Broyles ligament and the thick, poorly vascularized intermediate lamina of the thyroid cartilage[30,33–35] (**Fig. 4**).

At the anterior commissure, Broyles ligament is met by the insertional fibers of the vocalis muscle; at this muscular attachment point, the thyroid cartilage is devoid of a true inner perichondrium[32] (**Fig. 5**). Although Broyles ligament serves as the inner perichondrium at the anterior commissure, it is not as effective of a barrier to tumor invasion as a true intact perichondrium. In addition, ossification preferentially occurs at muscular attachment points. Ossification not only facilitates tumor invasion but, at the anterior commissure, the sclerotic process allows blood vessels adjacent to Broyles ligament to penetrate the thyroid cartilage creating a connection between the internal and external laryngeal blood supply further increasing the vulnerability to tumor spread[32,36] (see **Fig. 5**).

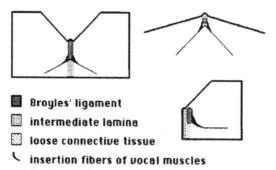

- ▨ **Broyles' ligament**
- ▦ **intermediate lamina**
- ▨ **loose connective tissue**
- ↖ **insertion fibers of vocal muscles**

Fig. 4. This graphic depicts the relationship of the vocal ligament tendon (Broyles' ligament), the intermediate lamina of the thyroid cartilage, and the insertional fibers of the vocal ligament. Note the loose connective tissue inferior to Broyles' ligament marks an area vulnerable to tumor invasion. (*From* Rucci L, Gammarota L, Cirri Borghi MB. Carcinoma of the anterior commissure of the larynx: I embryological and anatomic. Ann Otol Rhinol Laryngol 1996;105(4):303–8; with permission.)

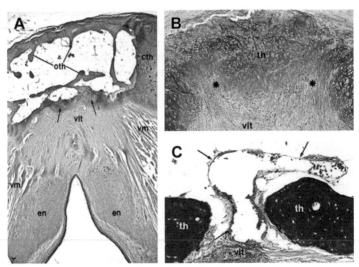

Fig. 5. (*A*) Micrograph through the anterior commissure showing an ossified thyroid carti-lage at the insertion of the vocal ligament tendons (Broyles ligament) with surrounding normal cartilage. Note the focal absence of a perichondrium at Broyles ligament (*arrow*) (to-luidine blue, original magnification ×30). (*B*) Micrograph through the insertion of the vocal ligament tendon (Broyles ligament). Collagen of Broyles ligament passes directly into the hyaline cartilage of the thyroid lamina. Perichondrium is absent at the area of the inser-tional fibers (*asterisk*) (Goldner staining, original magnification ×30). (*C*) Micrograph through the larynx at the level of the anterior commissure. Note the ossified cartilage with a blood vessel linking the internal and external laryngeal blood supply (*arrow*) (azan, original magnification ×372). cth, cartilaginous thyroid cartilage; en, elastic nodule; oth, ossified thyroid cartilage; th, ossified thyroid cartilage; vlt, vocal ligament tendon; vm, vocalis muscle. (*Adapted from* Paulsen F, Kimpel M, Lockemann U, et al. Effects of ageing on the insertion zones of the human vocal fold. J Anat 2000;196:41–54; with permission.)

Chemical Activators

Tumor growth requires the formation of new capillaries, and normally tumor capillary formation is initiated by when host vessels penetrate and feed the tumor. This process is initiated when the tumor releases the tumor angiogenesis factor. Brem and Folk-man[16] have shown that cartilage can inhibit the induction of capillary proliferation, sug-gesting the presence of a cartilage-mediated inhibition of tumor angiogenesis factor.[15,16]

As mentioned previously, collagenase activity is known to be associated with tumor growth and invasion. The enzymatic activity of collagenase is not secreted by the tu-mor itself, but rather it is activated by inflammation. The host tissue initiates a local in-flammatory response to the presence of a tumor, which is accentuated by the tumor's secretion of prostaglandin E2.[37] This focal inflammation stimulates the host stroma to produce activated collagenase, protease, and leucine aminopeptidase, which degrade tissue and break down the body's natural barriers to tumor spread.

Keratinizing tumors elicit a particularly strong inflammatory granulomatous reaction likely increasing the levels of proteolytic enzymes. Proteolytic enzymes preferentially cleave type IV collagen, a major structural component of the basement membrane, and thereby facilitate tumor invasion[8] (**Fig. 6**).

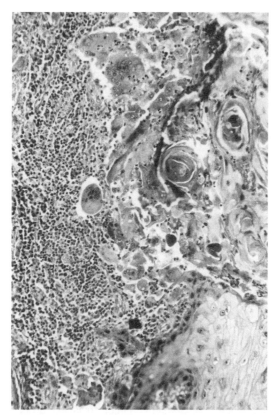

Fig. 6. Micrograph showing foreign body granulomatous reaction with giant cells surrounding keratinizing tumor (hematoxylin-eosin, original magnification ×325). (*From* Blitzer A. Regional behavioral variations of epidermoid carcinoma of the head and neck: a study in an animal model. Laryngoscope 1982;92(11):1219–38; with permission.)

Unlike collagenase, significant levels of elastase have not been found to be associated with carcinoma owing to the relative resistance to tumor invasion of arteries and other membranous structures that are rich in elastic fibers.[8]

SUMMARY

The barriers to tumor spread within the larynx are a product of laryngeal development, anatomic barriers, and enzymatic activity. Observational and histologic studies of the larynx have enabled us to reveal focal anatomic areas that are vulnerable to invasion. In addition, the enzymatic interplay between the tumor and the host tissue is an important factor to the spread of laryngeal tumor. Understanding laryngeal embryology, anatomy, and biology has helped us understand the propensity for local, regional, and distant spread of laryngeal carcinoma.

REFERENCES

1. Cooper MH. Anatomy of the larynx. In: Blitzer A, Brin MF, Ramig LO, editors. Neurologic disorders of the larynx. New York: Thieme; 2009. p. 3–9.

2. Tucker JA, Tucker ST. Posterior commissure of the human larynx revisited. J Voice 2010;24(3):252–9.
3. Reidenbach MM. The periepiglottic space: topographic relations and histological organization. J Anat 1996;188:173–82.
4. Sanders I, Wu BL, Mu L, et al. The innervation of the human posterior cricoarytenoid muscle: evidence for at least two neuromuscular compartments. Laryngoscope 1994;104(7):880–4.
5. Hirano M. Structure and vibratory behavior of the vocal folds. In: Sawashima M, Cooper FS, editors. Dynamic aspects of speech production. Tokyo: University of Tokyo Press; 1977. p. 13–27.
6. Porter PW, Vilenksy JA. The laryngeal saccule: clinical significance. Clin Anat 2012;25:647–9.
7. Hajek M. Anatomische Untesuchungen uber das Larynxodem. Arch Klin Chir 1891;42:46–93.
8. Blitzer A. Regional behavioral variations of epidermoid carcinoma of the head and neck: a study in an animal model. Laryngoscope 1982;92(11):1219–38.
9. Pressman J, Dowdy A, Libby R, et al. Further studies upon the submucosal compartments and lymphatics of the larynx by injection of dyes and radioisotopes. Ann Otol Rhinol Laryngol 1956;65:963–80.
10. Armstrong WB, Netterville JL. Anatomy of the larynx, trachea, and bronchi. Otolaryngol Clin North Am 1995;28:685–99.
11. Frazer E. The development of the larynx. J Anat Physiol 1909;44:156.
12. Tucker GF, Smith HR. A histological demonstration of the development of laryngeal connective tissue compartments. Trans Am Acad Ophthalmol Otolaryngol 1962;66:308–18.
13. Beitler JJ, Mahadeuia PS, Silver CE, et al. New barriers to ventricular invasion in paraglottic laryngeal cancer. Cancer 1994;73(10):2648–52.
14. Young N, Abdelmessih MW, Sasaki C. Hajek revisited: a histological examination of the quadrangular membrane. Ann Otol Rhinol Laryngol 2014;123(11): 765–8.
15. Gallo A, Morcetti P, De Vincentiis M, et al. Neoplastic infiltration of laryngeal cartilages: histocytochemical study. Laryngoscope 1992;102:891–5.
16. Brem H, Folkman J. Inhibition of tumor angiogenesis mediated by cartilage. J Exp Med 1975;141:427–39.
17. Takigawa M, Pan HO, Enomoto M, et al. A clonal human chondrosarcoma cell line produces an anti-angiogenic antitumor factor. Anticancer Res 1990;10(2A):311–5.
18. Takigawa M, Shirai E, Enomoto M, et al. Cartilage-derived anti-tumor factor (CATF) inhibits the proliferation of endothelial cells in culture. Cell Biol Int Rep 1985;9(7):619–25.
19. Takigawa M, Shirai E, Enomoto M, et al. A factor in conditioned medium of rabbit costal chondrocytes inhibits the proliferation of cultured endothelial cells and angiogenesis induced by B16 melanoma: its relation with cartilage-derived anti-tumor factor (CATF). Biochem Int 1987;14(2):357–63.
20. Pauli BU, Memoli VA, Kuettner KE. Regulation of tumor invasion by cartilage derived anti-invasion factor in vitro. J Natl Cancer Inst 1981;67(1):65–73.
21. Suzuki F. Cartilage-derived growth factor and antitumor factor: past, present, and future studies. Biochem Biophys Res Commun 1999;259(1):1–7.
22. Yeager VL, Archer CR. Anatomical routes for cancer invasion of laryngeal cartilages. Laryngoscope 1982;92(4):449–52.
23. Broyles EN. The anterior commissure tendon. Ann Otol Rhinol Laryngol 1943;52: 342–5.

24. Bagatella F, Bignardi L. Behavior of cancer at the anterior commissure of the larynx. Laryngoscope 1983;93(3):353–6.
25. Zbfiren P, Becket M, Ling H. Staging of laryngeal cancer: endoscopy, computed tomography and magnetic resonance versus histopathology. Eur Arch Otorhinolaryngol 1997;254(Suppl.1):S 117–22.
26. Becker M. Neoplastic invasion of laryngeal cartilage: radiologic diagnosis and therapeutic implications. Eur J Radiol 2000;33(3):216.
27. Pittam MR, Carter RL. Framework invasion by laryngeal carcinomas. Head Neck Surg 1982;4(3):200–8.
28. Gregor R, Hammond K. Framework invasion by laryngeal carcinoma. Am J Surg 1987;154:452–8.
29. Barnes L. Diseases of the larynx, hypopharynx, and trachea. In: Barnes L, editor. Surgical pathology of the head and neck. New York: Informa Healthcare; 2009. p. 109–200.
30. Rucci L, Gammarota L, Cirri Borghi MB. Carcinoma of the anterior commissure of the larynx: I embryological and anatomic. Ann Otol Rhinol Laryngol 1996;105(4):303–8.
31. Rucci L, Gammarota L, Oreste G. Carcinoma of the anterior commissure of the larynx: II proposal of a new staging. Ann Otol Rhinol Laryngol 1996;105(5):391–6.
32. Paulsen F, Kimpel M, Lockemann U, et al. Effects of ageing on the insertion zones of the human vocal fold. J Anat 2000;196:41–54.
33. Kirchner JA, Fischer J. Anterior commissure cancer- a clinical and laboratory study of 39 cases. Can J Otolaryngol 1975;4:637–43.
34. Kirchner JA. Invasion of the framework by laryngeal cancer. Acta Otolaryngol 1984;97:392–7.
35. Kirchner JA, Carter D. Intralaryngeal barriers to the spread of cancer. Acta Otolaryngol 1987;103:503–13.
36. Ambrosch P, Fazel A. Functional organ preservation in laryngeal and hypopharyngeal cancer. GMS Curr Top Otorhinolaryngol Head Neck Surg 2011;10:1–31.
37. Bennett A, Carter RL, Stamford IF, et al. Prostaglandin-like material extracted from squamous cell carcinomas of the head and neck. Br J Cancer 1980;41:204–8.

Evaluation of the Dysphonic Patient (in: Function Preservation in Laryngeal Cancer)

Chad W. Whited, MD[a], Seth H. Dailey, MD[b],*

KEYWORDS

- Diagnosis • Dysphonia • Hoarseness • Voice • Cancer • Laryngoscopy
- Stroboscopy

KEY POINTS

- Evaluation of the dysphonic patient begins as soon as the clinician can hear the patient's voice. This evaluation involves a thorough history, head and neck examination, a perceptual evaluation of the voice, and a detailed assessment of the patient's laryngeal anatomy and function.
- Dysphonia results from a disruption in the anatomy and function of the vocal folds. Stroboscopy is critical in evaluating the function of the vocal fold vibratory characteristics.
- High-speed digital imaging also can play an important role in patients with aperiodic vocal fold vibration.
- Concerning lesions warrant a biopsy for pathologic diagnosis.
- In the operating room, a telescope or microscope provides optimal visualization, mapping ability, and tactile evaluation of the tissue. Additionally, in-office biopsy is a cost-reducing and effective alternative in select patients for pathologic sampling.

INTRODUCTION

Dysphonia is defined as an impairment of the speaking or singing voice, and it affects up to one-third of people during their lifetime.[1,2] The evaluation of dysphonia by general otolaryngologists varies with different practice patterns depending on

Neither C.W. Whited nor S.H. Dailey have any conflicts of interest, financial or otherwise, to disclose.
[a] Otolaryngology-Head & Neck Surgery, University of Wisconsin at Madison, 600 Highland Avenue, BX7375 Clinical Science Cntr-H4, Madison, WI 53792-3284, USA; [b] Section of Laryngology and Voice Surgery, Otolaryngology-Head & Neck Surgery, University of Wisconsin at Madison, 600 Highland Avenue, BX7375 Clinical Science Cntr-H4, Madison, WI 53792-3284, USA
* Corresponding author.
E-mail address: Dailey@surgery.wisc.edu

Otolaryngol Clin N Am 48 (2015) 547–564
http://dx.doi.org/10.1016/j.otc.2015.04.003
0030-6665/15/$ – see front matter © 2015 Elsevier Inc. All rights reserved.

oto.theclinics.com

Abbreviations

CAPE-V	Consensus Auditory Perceptual Evaluation of Voice
DL	Direct laryngoscopy
F_o	Fundamental frequency
GRBAS	Grade, roughness, breathiness, asthenia, strain
HSDI	High-speed digital imaging
NBI	Narrow Band Imaging
SLP	Speech-Language Pathologist(s)
VHI	Voice Handicap Index
V-RQOL	Voice-related quality of life

training background, practice type, and available resources.[3] There are multiple techniques to visualize the larynx from mirror laryngoscopy to high-speed digital imaging (HSDI). Some practices frequently employ speech-language pathologists (SLPs) to assess the perceptual, aerodynamic, and acoustic measurements, as well as treatment counseling and therapy. This lack of consensus in approach to dysphonia contributed to the Academy of Otolaryngology–Head and Neck Surgery to develop clinical practice guidelines on dysphonia.[4] There are both benign and malignant factors that can cause dysphonia, but what is concerning is that up to 52% of patients with laryngeal cancer thought their hoarseness was harmless, leading to a delay in evaluation and treatment.[5] The guidelines list comorbidities that should trigger a patient and clinician to suspect a serious underlying cause of the dysphonia (**Box 1**). This article builds on the invaluable article by Blitzer, elsewhere in this issue, regarding laryngeal anatomy and function, and presents a laryngologist's focus on the different tools, highlights, and pitfalls in the evaluation of the dysphonic patient.

Box 1
Concerning signs with dysphonia

Conditions leading to suspicion of a "serious underlying cause"

Hoarseness with a history of tobacco or alcohol use

Hoarseness with concomitant discovery of a neck mass

Hoarseness after trauma

Hoarseness associated with hemoptysis, dysphagia, odynophagia, otalgia, or airway compromise

Hoarseness with accompanying neurologic symptoms

Hoarseness with unexplained weight loss

Hoarseness that is worsening

Hoarseness in an immunocompromised host

Hoarseness and possible aspiration of a foreign body

Hoarseness in a neonate

Unresolving hoarseness after surgery (intubation or neck surgery)

From Schwartz S, Cohen S, Dailey S, et al. Clinical practice guideline: hoarseness (dysphonia). Otolaryngol Head Neck Surg 2009;141(3 Suppl 2):S1–31; with permission.

HISTORY

Often clinicians have a referring diagnosis or physical examination finding from a colleague to guide an evaluation. However, referring diagnoses are commonly inaccurate, and a myopic evaluation can overlook findings that may influence treatment. The differential diagnosis for dysphonia is extensive (**Box 2**), and a thoughtful history can direct testing, treatment, and prognosis counseling. Therefore, the first part of any evaluation is a thorough and complete history. Elements include standard concerning signs and symptoms regarding pain, weight loss, and neck masses. Inquiring about cigarette smoking and alcohol consumption are crucial, as both are well-established risks factors for both laryngeal cancer and dysphonia.[6] With the dysphonic patient, additional details must be investigated. History of prior intubations, neck surgery, radiation, or trauma can all affect vocal quality. Upper aerodigestive tract diseases, such as gastroesophageal reflux disease, asthma, allergies, sinusitis, and inhaler use, can all contribute to dysphonia. A surgeon must consider the larynx in terms of its 3 main roles: voice, breathing, and swallowing. Evaluating one without the others can lead to incomplete decision-making.

Similar to the evaluation of pain, a surgeon must evaluate all of the aspects associated with the dysphonic complaint, including onset, duration, quality, frequency, severity, and alleviating and aggravating factors. Gradual onset can often imply a functional dysphonia or a small growing lesion. Abrupt onset is often associated with a hemorrhagic polyp or an acute injury. An onset associated with endotracheal tube intubation or anterior neck or thoracic operation could implicate an injury to the cricoarytenoid joint or vagus/recurrent laryngeal nerves. Persistent dysphonia after an upper respiratory tract infection could suggest a nerve paresis or residual inflammatory changes.

When a physician asks a patient about his or her voice, the common response is "it's just hoarse" or "it doesn't sound like my normal voice." Asking the patient to describe the nature of the vocal complaints without using the term "hoarse" can elucidate what it is exactly about the voice that is causing distress. Descriptors such as effortful, weak, short of breath, sore, lower pitch, or poor clarity are all part of a medical vernacular that a surgeon can use to narrow the differential diagnoses. A "breathy" or "effortful" voice is often due to incomplete closure of the vocal folds during phonation. Specific examples might include unilateral vocal fold paralysis or paresis, fixation from tumor invasion of the thyroarytenoid muscle or cricothyroid joint, vocal fold atrophy in presbylarynges, or a large posterior granuloma impeding closure. A "rough" or "strained" voice might be attributable to irregular vocal fold oscillation during phonation due to glottic asymmetry. Pathologies that could lead to roughness include muscle tension dysphonia, vocal fry, benign vocal lesions, anterior glottic web, neoplasm, leukoplakia, or vocal fold scar.

It is useful to evaluate the variability of the dysphonia and its pattern throughout the day. A voice that is consistently dysphonic with little fluctuating could implicate a constant anatomic abnormality. If a patient describes a period of normalcy surrounded by the dysphonic voice, this could represent a fluctuating nonorganic etiology, such as muscle tension dysphonia. An overall decline raises concern for a progressing neoplasm.

It is important to inquire about voice demands at work as well as previous vocal training. This may uncover compounding factors, such as fume or allergen exposure, or unhealthy vocal demands at a construction site, hair salon, or a large classroom. A patient's vocal experience also can guide the specificity of pretreatment counseling on vocal expectations, treatment decisions, and the extensiveness of posttreatment voice therapy.

Box 2
Differential diagnosis for dysphonia

Differential diagnosis dysphonia

Laryngitis

 Chronic

 Viral

 Bacterial

 Fungal

 Allergic

 Reflux

 Sicca

Benign lesions

 Polyp

 Varices

 Cyst

 Pseudocyst

 Nodules

 Granuloma

 Reinke edema

 Reactive lesion

 Hemorrhage

 Laryngocele

Airway stenosis

Web

Scar

Presbylarynges/Atrophy

Muscle tension dysphonia

Neurologic and neuromuscular

 Vocal fold paralysis

 Vocal fold paresis

 Spasmodic dystonia

 Tremor

 Clonus

 Cerebral vascular accident

 Parkinson disease

 Amyotrophic lateral sclerosis

 Myasthenia gravis

Recurrent respiratory papillomatosis

Leukoplakia

Neoplasm

 Verrucous

Squamous cell

Granular cell

Metastatic

Systemic disease

Rheumatologic lesions

Systemic lupus erythematosus

Sarcoidosis

Granulomatosis with polyangitis (Wegener)

Amyloidosis

Tuberculosis

Hypothyroidism

Syphilis

Polychondritis

Laryngeal trauma

Cricoarytenoid dislocation

Cricoarytenoid fixation

Vocal fold tear

A thorough history includes a review of past medical history, operations, and medications. Progressive neurologic diseases, such as tremor, Parkinson disease, and amyotrophic lateral sclerosis, all involve the larynx and voice in different forms. Upper and lower airway disease could lead to chronic inflammation from post nasal drip, productive pulmonary secretions, or chronic throat clearing. Previous anterior cervical surgeries, such as anterior cervical discectomy and fusion, thyroidectomy, or carotid endarterectomy, all place the recurrent laryngeal nerve and external branch of the superior laryngeal nerve at risk for injury with subsequent dysphonia. Previous intubations can lead to paresis, paralysis, arytenoid immobility, or granuloma. Medications can produce a rough voice, as is often a result from the drying effects of diuretics. Angiotensin-converting enzyme inhibitors have the well-known side effect of cough, which can lead to chronic irritation and dysphonia.

OFFICE EXAMINATION

Performer and music teacher Manuel Patricio Garcia of Spain first introduced the mirror laryngoscopy. It was subsequently adapted to the medical profession with modifications by Turk and Czermak.[7] A thorough mirror examination has often been the combination of art and science, and culminates as a rite of passage or clinical diagnostic skill exclusive to otolaryngologists. With the tongue drawn forward, the patient phonates "e" to elevate the larynx and protrude the base of tongue anteriorly for optimal viewing of the endolarynx.[8] Although the mirror provides a convenient and inexpensive examination, there are well-known limitations. It lacks magnification for finer lesions, anterior glottic visualization can be difficult, and the inability to record examinations limits patient education and review capabilities. The mirror laryngoscopy also precludes performing most voice tasks during the examination.

Rigid endoscopy is performed by placing a Hopkins rod through the mouth to the posterior oropharynx. Topical anesthesia may be needed to reduce the gag reflex. The Hopkins rod has an alternating air-lens system that permits transmission of the image from the distal to the proximal end with minimal distortion. The distal end of the rod has an angled lens, typically 70° or 90°, to permit a view of the inferiorly situated larynx. The endoscope is coupled to a high-intensity light source while relaying a magnified image to the proximal eyepiece. The rod also can be coupled to a stroboscopic light source or a high-speed digital camera (see later in this article). The naked eye can be used through the eyepiece, or a video-capturing device can be attached to the eyepiece for recording and reviewing of images later. The technique is similar to the mirror examination in that the patient is in the seated sniffing position with the tongue drawn forward. The rigid endoscope enables the physician to acquire high-quality images and detect the subtlest abnormalities. Similar to the mirror examination, the rigid examination limits the voice tasks, such as connected speech, because the device is occupying the oral cavity.

In a direct comparison between mirror laryngoscopy and rigid angled indirect laryngoscopy, the use of the rigid endoscope produced significantly less gagging and pain for the patient.[9] In addition, the rigid endoscope provided a more complete examination when compared with the mirror laryngoscopy, especially of the anterior glottis.

Fiberoptic flexible laryngoscopy involves using a small-diameter cable with optical fibers that transmit both light from the proximal source and the image from the distal target. Similar to the rigid endoscope, the eyepiece may be used with the naked eye or connected to an image-capturing device for recording and review. Unique to the flexible scope is that it passes through the nasal cavity, nasopharynx, and oropharynx, limiting the gag reflex. Topical nasal anesthesia is sometimes used for this examination, although its use has not been demonstrated to significantly reduce patients' discomfort.[10] Initially, these scopes were plagued with poor light intensity and image quality, making them substandard to rigid endoscopic examination. However, flexible endoscopes with small cameras placed at the distal tip of the scope have enhanced image resolution that is of essentially the same quality as rigid endoscopes. The advantages of flexible laryngoscopy include the ability to evaluate the palatal function, as well as a full range of connected speech, breathing, and singing tasks. The smaller sizes also allow pediatric laryngeal evaluation. Regular white light laryngoscopy is excellent at identifying lesions, but lacks the ability to assess the vibratory characteristics. Fortunately, stroboscopy also can be performed via flexible examination.

Stroboscopy uses a strobe light source synchronized to the vibratory frequency of the vocal folds to provide an image that appears to be still or in slow motion, depending on the settings selected. This uses the phenomena of flicker-free perception of light and the apparent motion from individual images.[11] As mentioned, either rigid or flexible endoscopes can be used to perform stroboscopy. The technique relies on the ability to capture the frequency of the patient with either a microphone or electroglottographic transducer and synchronize it with that strobe light source. Exact frequency synchronization provides what appears as a still image from a single point in the vibratory cycle. Quasi-synchronization (1–2 Hz above frequency) provides an image that appears to be in continuous motion of successive points in the vibratory cycle, giving the appearance of a slow-motion vibratory cycle. This feature allows detailed evaluation of the vibratory cycle and the viscoelastic properties of the mucosal vocal folds as the body-cover relationship can be inspected for any alteration. Vocal fold vibratory characteristics have been demonstrated to be critical in evaluating voice disorders, as the use of videostroboscopy leads to a change in treatment decisions in 14% to 33% of patients.[12–14] As mentioned, videostroboscopy relies on the ability to capture and synchronize with the patient's frequency. Patients with aperiodic vibratory cycles are unable to be synchronized with stroboscopy. Stroboscopy is ineffective at evaluating voice onset and offset, as a small amount of time is needed to synchronize before image production.

There are different aspects of the vocal folds that can be evaluated with videostroboscopy. One of the most recent and popular rating systems listed here provides a framework by which examinations can be evaluated in a systematic manner (**Fig. 1**).[15] The rater is asked to evaluate amplitude, vertical level match, mucosal wave, and the nonvibratory portion of the musculomembranous portion of the vocal fold. Supraglottic activity can be measured in a medial-to-lateral and an anterior-to-posterior compression pattern. The vocal fold edge is evaluated by both smoothness and straightness. Phase closure rates the percentage of time the vibratory cycle is in

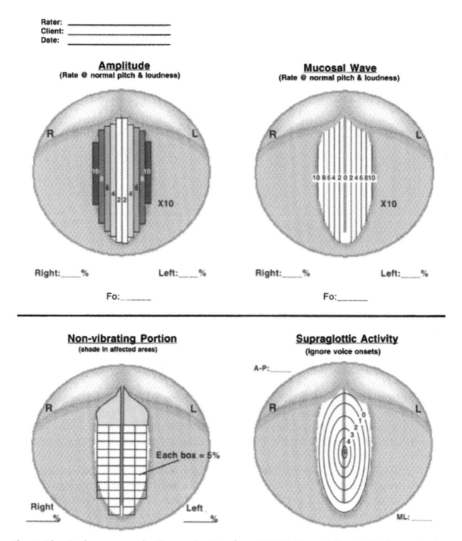

Fig. 1. The stroboscopy evaluation and rating form (SERF). (*From* Poburka BJ. A new stroboscopy rating form. J Voice 1999;13(3):403–13; with permission.)

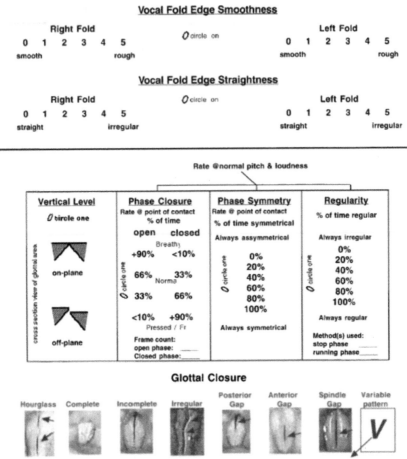

Fig. 1. (*continued*).

the closed or open phase, whereas phase symmetry rates the percentage of time the mucosal vibration is in symmetric phase. Regularity measures the percentage of time that one vibratory cycle is like the next. Glottal closure describes the quality or characteristic of the glottal closure pattern.

Videostroboscopy allows for a more detailed functional and anatomic evaluation of the vocal folds and their vibratory viscoelastic characteristics. Stroboscopy can reveal benign, premalignant, and malignant epithelial changes; however, it has been unable to consistently differentiate among these lesions based on vibratory characteristics alone.[16,17]

High-speed digital imaging may have utility beyond stroboscopy in the evaluation of vibratory properties of the vocal folds (**Fig. 2**).[18] It uses a rigid endoscope similar to rigid videostroboscopy, but instead of giving the illusion of glottal cycle frame-by-frame examination, HSDI captures images at the rate of 2000 to 5000 frames per second.[19] This allows for onset and offset examination, as well as patients with an aperiodic vibratory cycle or frequency fluctuation. Based on computer memory limitations, only approximately 2 to 8 seconds of phonation is recorded; however, this

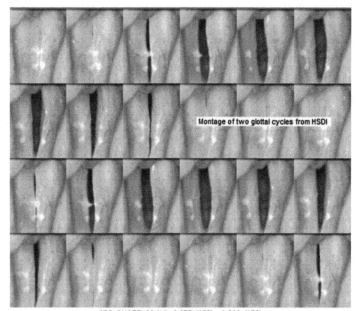

Montage of two glottal cycles from HSDI

SPC_SHORT_20.AVI: 0.077s(156) – 0.089s(179)

Fig. 2. HSDI. Montage from high-speed video at 2000 frames per second. (*From* Krausert CR, Olszewski AE, Taylor LN, et al. Mucosal wave measurement and visualization techniques. J Voice 2011;25(4):395–405; with permission.)

provides thousands of images. The frequency speed of image capturing can be increased as can the use of color imaging instead of black and white. However, both come with the trade-off of image quality. HSDI can be expensive and time-consuming; however, the quality of images and universal application to aperiodic voice pathologies make it clinically useful in certain scenarios.

The gold standard for laryngeal epithelial examination is still direct laryngoscopy (DL) in the operating room under general anesthesia. DL with a rigid endoscopic magnification allows for a close-up, magnified visual examination of the glottis. Angled endoscopes provide a refined examination of the ventricle, caudal surface of the vocal folds, the anterior commissure, the infraglottis, and the subglottis. Using the operating microscope frees up the surgeon's hands for precise palpation and proprioceptive examination of the entire vocal fold epithelium and body. These advantages allow an increased detection of rate of glottal lesions and altering the surgical plan.[20] Although DL is the gold standard, it is important to note that the larynges of all patients may not be able to be exposed in the operating room. Patients with trismus, an anterior larynx, postradiation neck changes, or previous cervical spinal pathology may still be best examined in the clinic or through a modified indirect approach in the operating room using a laryngeal mask anesthesia and flexible instrumentation.

Narrow band imaging (NBI) is another recent adjuvant to laryngeal examination. NBI applies a filtered light via flexible or rigid endoscope to the mucosa, highlighting the underlying superficial vasculature. Through filtering specific green and blue wavelengths corresponding to the peaks of hemoglobin absorption, the capillaries and superficial veins within the epithelium and lamina propria are enhanced.[21] NBI relies on the principle that neoplasms require neovascularization and, at the least, create a distortion of normal vascular patterns. These vascular pattern changes allow tumors to be detected when they otherwise would have been missed using traditional white light imaging (**Fig. 3**).[22] NBI has been demonstrated to enhance the sensitivity and accuracy of delineating suspicious lesions in the larynx.[23] Second, the borders between neoplasm and healthy epithelium are more distinguishable, aiding in preserving healthy mucosa during staging and treatment.[24]

VOICE EVALUATION MEASURES

Unfortunately, there is no "voice-o-gram" a clinician can use to quantitatively define the degree and quality of dysphonia in a fashion standardized across all patients. Therefore, we must rely on a combination of tools assessing psychosocial impact, perceptual analysis, acoustic analysis, and aerodynamic analysis (**Box 3**). This is important for many reasons, one of which is being able to compare outcome measures in the most patient-centered, meaningfully way possible.

PATIENT-BASED PSYCHOSOCIAL IMPACT

One way to evaluate dysphonia is by measuring its impact on a patient's quality of life. How dysphonia impacts a patient's function, activity performance, or role in society touches on the World Health Organization's International Classification of Impairments, Disabilities, and Handicaps. Multiple instruments have been founded and validated based on this approach to quality of life including the Voice Handicap Index (VHI), VHI-10, Voice-Related Quality of Life (V-RQOL), Voice Outcome Survey, Voice Activity and Participation Profile, and Voice Symptom Scale.[25]

The VHI is a 30-item questionnaire designed to examine the psychosocial consequences of voice disorders (**Table 1**).[26] This is broken down into emotional, physical, and functional responses to dysphonia with an 18-point difference representing a significant shift in impact. Another quality-of-life assessment tool is the V-QROL, which includes a physical component score and a mental component score.[27] Both the VHI and V-RQOL have been validated and used by many investigators to evaluate dysphonia in relation to laryngeal cancer and treatment outcomes.[28–32]

AUDITORY PERCEPTUAL MEASURES

Perceptual measures rely on the human auditory processing to make judgments of a patient's voice. It is exactly this perceptual change that often brings patients into the physician's office to be evaluated. Perceptual analysis should be an instantaneous

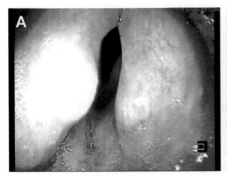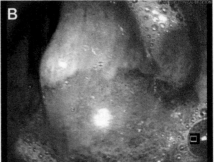

Fig. 3. (*A*) An in-office flexible endoscopic examination using white light. (*B*) An in-office flexible endoscopic examination using NBI. NBI demonstrates enhanced visualization of vascular stippling in neoplastic aryepiglottic fold mucosa.

Box 3
Voice evaluation measures (psychosocial, perceptual, acoustic, aerodynamic)

Psychosocial impact

Voice Handicap Index (VHI)

VHI 10

Voice-Related Quality of Life (V-RQOL)

Voice Activity and Participation Profile

Voice Outcomes Survey

Voice Symptom Scale (VoiSS)

Singing VHI

Perceptual analysis

"Severity, Roughness, Breathiness, Strain, Pitch, Loudness, Resonance, Tension, Fry, Breaks"

Grade, roughness, breathiness, asthenia, strain (GRBAS)

Consensus Auditory Perceptual Evaluation of Voice (CAPE-V)

Buffalo III Voice Profile

Stockholm Voice Evaluation Approach

Voice Profile Analysis

Acoustic analysis

Fundamental frequency

Intensity

Voice range profile

Spectography and spectral measures

Perturbation

Nonlinear measures

Aerodynamic analysis

Volume: maximum phonation time (MPT)

Airflow

Pressure: phonation threshold pressure, offset pressure, resistance

---

and continuous process of the physician's examination and evaluation. However, perceptual scoring is plagued with difficulties and inconsistencies given the reliance on the evaluator's subjective interpretation, experience, and vocabulary. This subjective quality makes perceptual measures as much of an art as it is a science.[33] Despite its limitations, perceptual analysis has its role in the clinical evaluation of a patient and outcomes measurements. Grade, roughness, breathiness, asthenia, strain (GRBAS) is a protocol rated on a 0 to 3-point scale for each measure, with the higher the score, the worse the perceptual effect.[34] The Consensus Auditory Perceptual Evaluation of Voice (**Fig. 4**) (CAPE-V) was developed by the American Speech-Language Hearing Association with the intention of improving consistency across practitioner evaluations.[35,36] CAPE-V evaluates severity, roughness, breathiness, strain, pitch, and loudness on a 100-mm analogue visual scale to be completed after standardized voice tasks. Studies have demonstrated slightly improved rater reliability with the CAPE-V,

Table 1
VHI Questionnaire

PART I: Functional aspect

1. Do people have difficulty understanding your voice?	0 1 2 3 4
2. Do people have difficulty understanding you in noisy environments?	0 1 2 3 4
3. Does your family have difficulty hearing you when you call them at home?	0 1 2 3 4
4. Do you stop using the telephone because of your voice?	0 1 2 3 4
5. Do you avoid groups of people because of your voice?	0 1 2 3 4
6. Do you talk less to friends, neighbors and relatives because of your voice?	0 1 2 3 4
7. Do people ask you to repeat yourself when talking to you face-to-face?	0 1 2 3 4
8. Does your voice restrict you in your personal and social lives?	0 1 2 3 4
9. Do you feel left out in conversations or discussions because of your voice?	0 1 2 3 4
10. Has your voice problem caused you to lose your job?	0 1 2 3 4

PART II: Physical aspect

1. Do you feel breathless when talking?	0 1 2 3 4
2. Does your voice vary during the day?	0 1 2 3 4
3. Do people ask, "What's wrong with your voice?"	0 1 2 3 4
4. Does your voice feel hissy or dry?	0 1 2 3 4
5. Do you struggle to produce your voice?	0 1 2 3 4
6. Is the clarity of your voice unpredictable?	0 1 2 3 4
7. Do you try to change your voice to sound different?	0 1 2 3 4
8. Does it take a lot of effort to speak?	0 1 2 3 4
9. Is your voice worse at the end of the day?	0 1 2 3 4
10. Does your voice fail in the middle of a conversation?	0 1 2 3 4

PART III: Emotional aspect

1. Do you feel tense when talking to other people because of your voice?	0 1 2 3 4
2. Do people get irritated because of your voice?	0 1 2 3 4
3. Do you feel other people do not understand your voice problem?	0 1 2 3 4
4. Does your voice bother you?	0 1 2 3 4
5. Are you less sociable because of your voice?	0 1 2 3 4
6. Do you feel impaired because of your voice problem?	0 1 2 3 4
7. Do you dislike it when people ask you to repeat yourself?	0 1 2 3 4
8. Do you feel embarrassed when people ask you to repeat yourself?	0 1 2 3 4
9. Does your voice make you feel incompetent?	0 1 2 3 4
10. Do you feel ashamed of your voice problem?	0 1 2 3 4

0, Never; 1, Almost never; 2, Sometimes; 3, Almost always; 4, Always.

Courtesy of the American Speech-Language-Hearing Association, Rockville, MD; with permission.

relatively good reliability between GRBAS and CAPE-V, but weak agreement with patient-based questionnaires, such as V-QROL.[36,37]

ACOUSTIC MEASURES

Acoustic analysis is based on the source-filter theory of speech production, where the glottal spectrum sound source is then filtered into a modified output waveform.[38] As the glottal spectrum travels through the supralaryngeal cavity, individual

Consensus Auditory-Perceptual Evaluation of Voice (CAPE-V)

Name:_____   Date:_____

The following parameters of voice quality will be rated upon completion of the following tasks:
1. Sustained vowels, /a/ and /i/ for 3-5 seconds duration each.
2. Sentence production:
   a. The blue spot is on the key again.   d. We eat eggs every Easter.
   b. How hard did he hit him?   e. My mama makes lemon muffins.
   c. We were away a year ago.   f. Peter will keep at the peak.
3. Spontaneous speech in response to: "Tell me about your voice problem." or "Tell me how your voice is functioning."

> **Legend:**   C = Consistent   I = Intermittent
> MI = Mildly Deviant   MO = Moderately Deviant   SE = Severely Deviant
> Although the PDF scale is accurate, printer configurations vary. Verify that your paper copy has accurate 100-mm lines before reproducing this form.

Overall Severity _____   C   I   ___/100
                  MI   MO   SE

Roughness   _____   C   I   ___/100
                  MI   MO   SE

Breathiness   _____   C   I   ___/100
                  MI   MO   SE

Strain   _____   C   I   ___/100
                  MI   MO   SE

Pitch   (Indicate the nature of the abnormality): _____
                  _____   C   I   ___/100
                  MI   MO   SE

Loudness   (Indicate the nature of the abnormality): _____
                  _____   C   I   ___/100
                  MI   MO   SE

_____   _____   C   I   ___/100
                  MI   MO   SE

_____   _____   C   I   ___/100
                  MI   MO   SE

COMMENTS ABOUT RESONANCE: NORMAL   OTHER (Provide description):_____

_____

ADDITIONAL FEATURES (for example, diplophonia, fry, falsetto, asthenia, aphonia, pitch instability, tremor, wet/gurgly, or other relevant terms):

Clinician:_____

Fig. 4. Consensus auditory perceptual evaluation of voice. (The CAPE-V was developed by the American Speech-Language-Hearing Association's Special Interest Group 3 (formerly known as Special Interest Division 3), Voice and Voice Disorders, and is used and reproduced herein under license. © [2006, 2010] American Speech-Language-Hearing Association. All rights in and to the CAPE-V are reserved and held by the American Speech-Language-Hearing Association.)

frequency components are either maximized into formants or minimized. Different acoustic measures include fundamental frequency (F_o), perturbation indices (jitter and shimmer), nonlinear measures, voice range profiles, and spectral and cepstral measures.

F_o is determined by the vocal fold oscillation rate as measured in hertz (Hz). It is dependent on characteristics of the vocal folds themselves, including mass, length, and tension. Varying these variables changes the subsequent frequency of the voice. Children, with shorter and thinner folds, have an F_o of 220 to 240 Hz, which subsequently diverges in adulthood to a female range of 200 to 220 Hz or adult male range of 100 to 120 Hz.[39]

Vocal intensity, or loudness, as measured in decibels is a product of subglottic pressure and vocal fold vibratory amplitude. Changes in the ability to generate subglottic pressure, poor glottal valve competency, or viscoelastic properties changes that restrict mucosal excursion all result in reduced intensity.

The voice range profile, or phonetogram, is a visual representation of the relationship between intensity and pitch (**Fig. 5**). It represents the minimum and maximum of intensity and frequency, and there have been demonstrated restrictions and changes in the phonetogram after endoscopic cordectomy for glottic cancer.[40] The vocal range profile is something most patients often are not mindful of until it has been reduced from cancer or its subsequent treatment. Knowledge of it should guide the surgeon in counseling that posttreatment voice outcomes will be limited in range and intensity.

Spectography and cepstral-based measures estimate irregular formant patterns and voice disruption in continuous speech. A meta-analysis on acoustic measures and overall voice quality found the cepstral metric the most promising and robust acoustic measure to dysphonia severity.[41]

AERODYNAMIC MEASURES

Aerodynamic analysis of the voice involves measuring different quantitative values along the vocal tract. These include flow volume, maximum phonation time, phonation

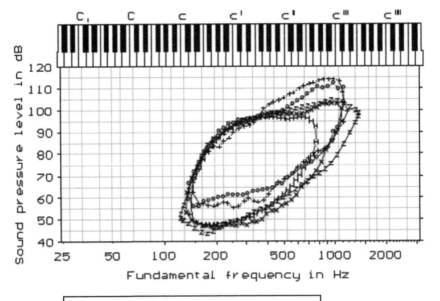

-+-+-+-	Professional soprano	
-H-H-H-	Teacher	
-o-o-o-	Professional mezzo soprano and soprano	
-x-x-x-	Untrained voices	
-z-z-z-	Trained voices	

Fig. 5. Phonetogram (Voice Range Profile [VRP]). A selection of average/norm VRP for the female voice. (*From* Pabon P, Stallinga R, Södersten M, et al. Effects on vocal range and voice quality of singing voice training: the classically trained female voice. J Voice 2014;28(1):36–51; with permission.)

threshold pressure and flow, and offset pressure. Increasing the area of endoscopic cordectomy increases phonation threshold pressure and flow rate, leading to a breathy and rough voice.[42] Also, increased phonation threshold pressure is correlated to increased vocal fatigue and effort.[43]

Briefly, it is important to emphasize the role of the SLP in laryngeal cancer. In addition to the collection and interpretation of the previously mentioned voice measures, the SLP provides expertise in posttreatment voice and swallowing rehabilitation.[44,45] The SLP provides an integral piece of the continuity of patient care, strengthening the relationship with the patient, and providing an extra resource the surgeon may not have time or the knowledge to fulfill.

DIAGNOSTIC SPECIMEN

The culmination of the evaluation of the dysphonic patient is the biopsy of any concerning lesions for pathologic diagnosis. Tissue diagnosis is required before any intervention of a presumed malignant lesion. Traditionally, this is performed in the operating room with the patient under general anesthesia with a DL. There are multiple descriptions of the proper technique for DL and an arsenal of laryngoscopes designed for unique scenarios.[46,47] The underlying principles are all the same. There must be a preoperative assessment of the anesthesia risks of the patient, including heart and lung disease. A surgeon must avoid injuring normal structures, such as teeth, lips, gums, tongue, and pharyngeal and laryngeal mucosa. One prospective study demonstrated a 37% risk of a minor complication after suspension laryngoscopy, including taste and swallowing disturbances, with the average effects lasting 11 days.[48] A DL consists of a thorough evaluation of all of the structures in the upper aerodigestive tract with biopsies of any concerning lesions. Although biopsies must be adequate for diagnosis, particularly on the vocal folds, they must all avoid injuring uninvolved epithelium and unnecessary subsequent permanent dysphonia. Overzealous biopsies or stripping run the risks of permanently damaging the viscoelastic properties of the lamina propria. Scar and sulcus formation of the epithelium can lead to permanent dysphonia that is difficult to rehabilitate. This caution must be viewed in light of the entire clinical picture given the severity or lack thereof in a patient's disease and their likely treatment pathway.

Another option that is emerging as a safe, effective, and cost-reducing method for obtaining permanent tissue diagnosis is the in-office biopsy.[49–51] In-office biopsy bypasses risks involved with anesthesia, negates the need to manage a difficult intubation, and reduces the overall cost of treatment. This report demonstrated that in-office biopsy reduces the cost of tissue diagnosis from approximately $9000 to $2000, while reducing the time to overall treatment from approximately 48 days to 24 days. Success from in-office biopsy ranges from 94% to 98%.

SUMMARY

Evaluation of the dysphonic patient begins as soon as the patient walks in the door with attentive listening of his or her voice and can lead all the way to the operating room, as appropriate. Training one's ear to appreciate the subtleties of voice characteristics will allow the physician to hone the pretest probability of a diagnosis before any laryngeal examination. The mirror laryngoscopy may be a convenient, initial examination; however, any patient with a persistent vocal complaint warrants a more detailed inspection of the vocal folds with a magnified, reviewable technique. There are multiple numerous voice evaluation measures, and their specific application value is still being determined. However, they do provide the clinician with objective measures by which to gauge and demonstrate the effects of treatment. The SLP is an important member of the treatment team, providing skills in voice evaluation, treatment counseling, and functional rehabilitation. Finally, for concerning or persistent lesions, biopsy, whether in the operating room or the office, provides the definitive diagnosis to guide subsequent counseling and treatment.

REFERENCES

1. American Speech-Language-Hearing Association. The use of voice therapy in the treatment of dysphonia [Technical Report]. 2005. Available at: www.asha.org/policy. Accessed September 15, 2014.
2. Roy N, Merrill RM, Gray SD, et al. Voice disorders in the general population: prevalence, risk factors, and occupational impact. Laryngoscope 2005;115:1988–95.
3. Cohen SM, Pitman MJ, Noordzij JP, et al. Management of dysphonic patients by otolaryngologists. Otolaryngol Head Neck Surg 2012;147(2):289–94.
4. Schwartz S, Cohen S, Dailey S, et al. Clinical practice guideline: hoarseness (dysphonia). Otolaryngol Head Neck Surg 2009;141(3 Suppl 2):S1–31.
5. Brouha XD, Tromp DM, de Leeuw JR, et al. Laryngeal cancer patients: analysis of patient delay at different tumor stages. Head Neck 2005;27:289–95.
6. Hashibe M, Boffetta P, Zaridze D, et al. Contribution of tobacco and alcohol to the high rates of squamous cell carcinoma of the supraglottis and glottis in Central Europe. Am J Epidemiol 2007;165(7):814–20.
7. Alberti PW. The history of laryngology: a centennial celebration. Otolaryngol Head Neck Surg 1996;114(3):345–54.
8. Benjamin B. Endolaryngeal surgery. 1st edition. London: The Livery House; 1998.
9. Dunklebarger J, Rhee D, Kim S, et al. Video rigid laryngeal endoscopy compared to laryngeal mirror examination: an assessment of patient comfort and clinical visualization. Laryngoscope 2009;119(2):269–71.
10. Sunkaraneni VS, Jones SE. Topical anaesthetic or vasoconstrictor preparations for flexible fibre-optic nasal pharyngoscopy and laryngoscopy. Cochrane Database Syst Rev 2011;(3):CD005606.
11. Mehta DD, Deliyski DD, Hillman RE. Commentary on why laryngeal stroboscopy really works: clarifying misconceptions surrounding Talbot's law and the persistence of vision. J Speech Lang Hear Res 2010;53(5):1263–7.
12. Sataloff RT, Speigel JR, Hawkshaw MJ. Strobovideolaryngoscopy: results and clinical value. Ann Otol Rhinol Laryngol 1991;100:725–7.
13. Casiano RR, Zaveri V, Lundy DS. Efficacy of videostroboscopy in the diagnosis of voice disorders. Otolaryngol Head Neck Surg 1992;107:95–100.
14. Woo P, Colton R, Casper J, et al. Diagnostic value of stroboscopic examination in hoarse patients. J Voice 1991;5:231–8.
15. Poburka BJ. A new stroboscopy rating form. J Voice 1999;13(3):403–13.
16. Colden D, Zeitels SM, Hillman RE, et al. Stroboscopic assessment of vocal fold keratosis and glottic cancer. Ann Otol Rhinol Laryngol 2001;110(4):293–8.
17. Djukic V, Milovanovic J, Jotic AD, et al. Stroboscopy in detection of laryngeal dysplasia effectiveness and limitations. J Voice 2014;28(2):262.
18. Krausert CR, Olszewski AE, Taylor LN, et al. Mucosal wave measurement and visualization techniques. J Voice 2011;25(4):395–405.
19. Jiang JJ, Yumoto E, Lin SJ, et al. Quantitative measurement of mucosal wave by high-speed photography in excised larynges. Ann Otol Rhinol Laryngol 1998;107:98–103.
20. Dailey SH, Spanou K, Zeitels S. The evaluation of benign glottic lesions: rigid telescopic stroboscopy versus suspension microlaryngoscopy. J Voice 2007;21(1):112–8.

21. Piazza C, Dessouky O, Peretti G, et al. Narrow-band imaging: a new tool for evaluation of head and neck squamous cell carcinomas. Review of the literature. Acta Otorhinolaryngol Ital 2008;28(2):49–54.
22. Lin YC, Wang WH, Lee KF, et al. Value of narrow band imaging endoscopy in early mucosal head and neck cancer. Head Neck 2012;34(11):1574–9.
23. Kraft M, Fostiropoulos K, Gürtler N, et al. Value of narrow band imaging in the early diagnosis of laryngeal cancer. Head Neck 2014. [Epub ahead of print].
24. Imaizumi M, Okano W, Tada Y, et al. Surgical treatment of laryngeal papillomatosis using narrow band imaging. Otolaryngol Head Neck Surg 2012;147(3):522–4.
25. Branski RC, Cukier-Blaj S, Pusic A, et al. Measuring quality of life in dysphonic patients: a systematic review of content development in patient-reported outcomes measures. J Voice 2010;24(2):193–8.
26. Jacobson B, Johnson A, Grywalski C, et al. The voice handicap index (VHI): development and validation. Am J Speech Lang Pathol 1997;6:66–70.
27. Hogikyan ND, Sethuraman G. Validation of an instrument to measure voice-related quality of life (V-RQOL). J Voice 1999;13(4):557–69.
28. Stewart MG, Chen AY, Stach CB. Outcomes analysis of voice and quality of life in patients with laryngeal cancer. Arch Otolaryngol Head Neck Surg 1998;124(2):143–8.
29. Cohen SM, Garrett CG, Dupont WD, et al. Voice-related quality of life in T1 glottic cancer: irradiation versus endoscopic excision. Ann Otol Rhinol Laryngol 2006;115(8):581–6.
30. Taylor SM, Kerr P, Fung K, et al. Treatment of T1b glottic SCC: laser vs. radiation—a Canadian multicenter study. J Otolaryngol Head Neck Surg 2013;42:22.
31. Fung K, Lyden TH, Lee J, et al. Voice and swallowing outcomes of an organ-preservation trial for advanced laryngeal cancer. Int J Radiat Oncol Biol Phys 2005;63(5):1395–9.
32. Oridate N, Homma A, Suzuki S, et al. Voice-related quality of life after treatment of laryngeal cancer. Arch Otolaryngol Head Neck Surg 2009;135(4):363–8.
33. Welham N. Clinical voice evaluation. In: Aronson AE, Bless D, editors. Clinical voice disorders. 4th edition. New York: Thieme; 2009. p. 134–66.
34. Hirano M. Clinical examination of voice. New York: Springer-Verlag; 1981.
35. Kempster GB, Gerratt BR, Verdolini Abbott K, et al. Consensus auditory-perceptual evaluation of voice: development of a standardized clinical protocol. Am J Speech Lang Pathol 2009;18(2):124–32.
36. Zraick RI, Kempster GB, Connor NP, et al. Establishing validity of the Consensus Auditory-Perceptual Evaluation of Voice (CAPE-V). Am J Speech Lang Pathol 2011;20(1):14–22.
37. Karnell MP, Melton SD, Childes JM, et al. Reliability of clinician-based (GRBAS and CAPE-V) and patient-based (V-RQOL and IPVI) documentation of voice disorders. J Voice 2007;21(5):576–90.
38. Fant G. Acoustic theory of speech production. Hague (The Netherlands): Mouton; 1960.
39. Brown WS Jr, Morris RJ, Hollien H, et al. Speaking fundamental frequency characteristics as a function of age and professional singing. J Voice 1991;5(4):310–5.
40. Bahannan AA, Slavíček A, Černý L, et al. Effectiveness of transoral laser microsurgery for precancerous lesions and early glottic cancer guided by analysis of voice quality. Head Neck 2014;36(6):763–7.
41. Maryn Y, Roy N, De Bodt M, et al. Acoustic measurement of overall voice quality: a meta-analysis. J Acoust Soc Am 2009;126(5):2619–34.

42. Mendelsohn AH, Xuan Y, Zhang Z. Voice outcomes following laser cordectomy for early glottic cancer: a physical model investigation. Laryngoscope 2014; 124(8):1882–6.
43. Chang A, Karnell MP. Perceived phonatory effort and phonation threshold pressure across a prolonged voice loading task: a study of vocal fatigue. J Voice 2004;18(4):454–66.
44. Miller S. The role of the speech-language pathologist in voice restoration after total laryngectomy. CA Cancer J Clin 1990;40(3):174–82.
45. Starmer HM, Gourin CG. Is speech language pathologist evaluation necessary in the nonoperative treatment of head and neck cancer? Laryngoscope 2013; 123(7):1571–2.
46. Zeitels SM, Burns JA, Dailey SH. Suspension laryngoscopy revisited. Ann Otol Rhinol Laryngol 2004;113(1):16–22.
47. Benjamin B, Lindholm CE. Systematic direct laryngoscopy: the Lindholm laryngoscopes. Ann Otol Rhinol Laryngol 2003;112(9 Pt 1):787–97.
48. Rosen CA, Andrade Filho PA, Scheffel L, et al. Oropharyngeal complications of suspension laryngoscopy: a prospective study. Laryngoscope 2005;115(9): 1681–4.
49. Naidu H, Noordzij JP, Samim A, et al. Comparison of efficacy, safety, and cost-effectiveness of in-office cup forcep biopsies versus operating room biopsies for laryngopharyngeal tumors. J Voice 2012;26(5):604–6.
50. Cohen JT, Safadi A, Fliss DM, et al. Reliability of a transnasal flexible fiberoptic in-office laryngeal biopsy. JAMA Otolaryngol Head Neck Surg 2013;139(4):341–5.
51. Lippert D, Hoffman MR, Dang P, et al. In-office biopsy of upper airway lesions: safety, tolerance, and effect on time to treatment. Laryngoscope 2015;125(4): 919–23.

Role of Advanced Laryngeal Imaging in Glottic Cancer

Early Detection and Evaluation of Glottic Neoplasms

Kathleen M. Tibbetts, MD, Melin Tan, MD*

KEYWORDS

- Glottic cancer • Laryngeal imaging • Videostroboscopy • High-speed imaging
- Videokymography • Optical coherence tomography • Autofluorescence
- Biologic endoscopy

KEY POINTS

- Direct laryngoscopy and biopsy are the gold standard for diagnosis of laryngeal cancer, but multiple imaging modalities exist and are in development that aid in the identification of early glottic neoplasms.
- Videostroboscopy, high-speed imaging, and videokymography characterize the vibratory properties of the vocal folds and can identify lesions that disrupt the normal mucosal wave.
- Optical coherence tomography, autofluorescence, and biologic endoscopy techniques noninvasively provide information about superficial and deep tissue structure.
- Computed tomographic scan, MRI, PET, and ultrasound can provide information relevant to staging of the primary tumor as well as about nodal metastases.

INTRODUCTION

Laryngeal carcinomas account for approximately 2.4% of new malignancies worldwide each year.[1] According to the American Cancer Society, 10,000 new cases of laryngeal cancer are diagnosed in the United States annually and result in 3900 yearly deaths.[2] More than 95% of laryngeal cancers are the squamous cell carcinoma (SCC) type.[3] The glottic larynx is the most common site of occurrence of laryngeal SCC.[4] Laryngeal cancers that are considered "early" typically include carcinoma in situ (CIS), T1, and T2 lesions without metastasis. In CIS, malignant cells are present but

The authors have no conflicts of interest to disclose.
Department of Otorhinolaryngology-Head and Neck Surgery, Montefiore Medical Center, Albert Einstein College of Medicine, 3400 Bainbridge Avenue, 3rd Floor, Bronx, NY 10467, USA
* Corresponding author.
E-mail address: mtangel@montefiore.org

Abbreviations	
AF	Autofluorescence
AFE	Autofluorescence endoscopy
AH	Acriflavine hydrochloride
ALA	Aminolevulinic acid
CE	Contact endoscopy
CEM	Confocal endomicroscopy
CIS	Carcinoma in situ
CT	Computed tomography
FDG	18F-fluorodeoxyglucose
HSI	High-speed imaging
NBI	Narrow band imaging
NPV	Negative predictive value
OCT	Optical coherence tomography
PPV	Positive predictive value
PS-OCT	Polarization sensitive optical coherence tomography
PTP	Fluorophore protoporphyrin IX
RS	Raman spectroscopy
SCC	Squamous cell carcinoma
SLP	Superficial lamina propria
US	Ultrasound
USPIO	Ultrasmall supramagnetic iron oxide

have not penetrated the basement membrane.[5] T1 lesions are limited to one (T1a) or both (T1b) vocal folds, with normal vocal fold mobility. T2 lesions extend to the supraglottis or subglottis and may impair vocal fold mobility without vocal fold fixation.

Early detection of pathologic tissue change is of utmost importance for effective treatment and the preservation of function in glottic malignancy. It can be difficult to find a balance between ensuring adequate resection and favorable oncologic outcome with preserving laryngeal structure and function. Imaging has traditionally been an important adjunct in the diagnosis, staging, and monitoring of glottic neoplasms. Although direct laryngoscopy and biopsy are the gold standard for definitive diagnosis of glottic cancers, radiologic imaging modalities have traditionally provided essential information regarding overall staging and prognosis, resectability, and the feasibility of subtotal surgical options.[6] Accurate identification of tumor margins within the larynx is also paramount to maximize oncologic outcome, because leaving positive margins increases the risk of local recurrence by 32% to 80%.[7] The goal of this article is to provide an overview of advanced techniques in laryngeal imaging and their application to the diagnosis, treatment, and long-term follow-up of glottic neoplasms.

INDIRECT LARYNGOSCOPY

Perhaps the most useful examination tool in the general otolaryngologic practice is indirect laryngoscopy, which can be performed by either laryngeal mirror examination or flexible fiber-optic endoscope. Irregularities of laryngeal mucosa may be concerning for malignancy. Because differentiating malignancy from benign processes is not predictable based on gross appearance, direct laryngoscopy and biopsy are warranted. However, the burning question in every patient's mind when they are diagnosed with a concerning laryngeal mass is what is the likelihood of malignancy. The largest study currently available evaluating clinical leukoplakia was performed by Isenberg and colleagues[8] in 2008 and combined their 15-year institutional experience with a review of the literature from the prior 50 years. They noted that there was no dysplasia in 54% of leukoplakias, mild to moderate dysplasia in 34%, and either CIS or SCC in 15%. SCC later developed in 4% of patients with no dysplasia at the time of biopsy, in 10% of patients with mild to moderate dysplasia at the time of biopsy, and in 18% with CIS at the time of biopsy. Although a general guideline can be elicited for patient counseling from these findings, all suspicious lesions require biopsy confirmation.

VIDEOSTROBOSCOPY

Videostroboscopy is a well-established method of imaging the vocal folds that allows the examiner to assess vocal fold vibration.[9] It is a noninvasive in-office examination that requires only occasional topical anesthesia, results in minimal patient discomfort, and is an integral part of the standard workup for dysphonia. A synchronized flashing light is directed onto the vocal folds via a rigid or flexible endoscope, effectively providing a still photo of the vocal folds in the midst of vibratory motion. By synchronizing the stroboscopic light to the frequency of the repetitive vocal fold vibration, the viewer perceives vocal fold vibration at a much slower rate than the actually vibratory speed. Videostroboscopy is a useful tool in the workup and diagnosis of hoarseness.[10,11] The visual effect of slower vocal fold oscillation is particularly helpful in the evaluation of abnormalities of laryngeal structure, vibratory asymmetry, and decreased or absent vibration.[12] It can also characterize abnormalities in glottic closure and allows measuring of glottal gap.[13–15] Stroboscopy has been shown to be able to accurately guide the diagnosis of benign midmembranous vocal fold lesions such as nodules, polyps, and cysts.[16] Because of its ability to detect variations in vocal fold vibration, videostroboscopy may be used to characterize vocal fold epithelial lesions. Vocal fold hyperkeratosis has been shown to decrease the amplitude and inhibit the mucosal wave of the vocal fold on videostroboscopic examination.[17] The mass effect on the vocal fold causes a lowered fundamental frequency. It has also been suggested that complete loss of vibration suggests early invasive carcinoma.[17] The vocal ligament and intermediate layer of the lamina propria are largely responsible for vocal fold vibration amplitude. Amplitude will be reduced as lesions become more infiltrative because the freedom of the epithelium to vibrate is compromised. Colden and colleagues,[18] however, showed that reduced amplitude of vocal fold vibration and mucosal wave propagation in vocal fold keratosis did not reliably predict the presence of malignancy or depth of invasion into the lamina propriae. They did suggest that an intact mucosal wave likely indicates that there is not extensive invasion into the vocal ligament. In reality, a cancerous lesion may demonstrate normal vibration amplitude and mucosal wave propagation if there is enough superficial lamina propria (SLP) underlying the lesion to allow for pliability of the epithelium. Alternatively, a lesion with normal amplitude and mucosal wave cannot be assumed to be benign. A benign lesion may cause a significant decrease in mucosal wave and amplitude perhaps because of compensatory phonotrauma confounding the examination. In addition, a cancerous lesion may cause complete loss of vibration and mucosal wave with no invasion into the vocal ligament. The ability of stroboscopy to detect abnormalities in the mucosal wave propagation, while not inherently diagnostic of malignancy, can alert the examiner of potentially cancerous lesions and lead to further workup.

HIGH-SPEED IMAGING

High-speed imaging (HSI) is a laryngeal imaging technique that allows for thousands of images of the vibrating vocal folds to be taken per second, usually via a rigid endoscope.[19] This technique overcomes some of the shortcomings of videostroboscopy, such as its dependence on periodic vibration and a minimum requisite phonation time of 2 seconds.[20] Because stroboscopy requires periodicity to produce the strobe effect, it cannot accurately reveal vibratory patterns in cases of dysphonia caused by aperiodic vibration.[21] HSI captures at least 2000 frames per second, or approximately10 to 20 frames per vibratory cycle depending on the fundamental frequency. Thus, it is not dependent on periodic vibratory motion and can reveal more about vibratory behavior than videostroboscopy.[22] For example, HSI has been shown to be able to detect subtle features that indicate vocal fold paresis that are not evident on fiber-optic laryngoscopy or videostroboscopy.[23] HSI is not yet widely available in clinical practice, however, and its practical applications continue to be defined. A study comparing the diagnostic accuracy of HSI compared with videostroboscopy found no difference between the 2 modalities in the diagnosis of 28 patients with dysphonia. The authors do, however, endorse the utility of HSI in challenging diagnostic cases such as vocal fold scar.[24] Other studies have shown HSI to be more accurate and interpretable than stroboscopy in patients with vocal pathologic abnormality resulting in aperiodic voices.[21,25,26] Patel and colleagues[21] advocate that in cases of severe dysphonia with values exceeding 0.87% jitter, 4.4% shimmer, and a signal-to-noise ratio of less than 15.4 dB on acoustic analysis, HSI may aid in clinic decision-making. Like stroboscopy, HSI does not directly diagnose malignant vocal fold lesions, but can detect subtle abnormalities in the mucosal vibratory properties that may spur further workup of potentially cancerous laryngeal lesions. An example of a series of images created with HSI in a patient with vocal fold scar is shown in **Fig. 1**.

VIDEOKYMOGRAPHY

Videokymography is an additional method to measure the vibratory capabilities of the vocal folds. Images from a single transverse line perpendicular to the glottal line are recorded, and successive images are shown in real-time on a monitor along with the time dimension. Once the pixel lines are extracted, they are configured consecutively side-by-side based on frame number to create a kymogram. The kymogram visualizes the motion of the mucosal wave, displaying the open and closed phases, periodicity, left to right symmetry, phase difference, and amplitude.[27] Thus videokymography allows for the assessment of left to right asymmetries, open quotient, and propagation of mucosal waves. Both standard and high-speed modes are available, with the former capturing 50 to 60 images per second, and the latter providing nearly 8000 images per second.[19] The earliest videokymography systems were only capable of generating one kymogram per examination.[28,29] In addition, because the scanning camera uniquely displayed time on one axis and the single line of the video image on another axis, the 2-dimensional video imaging of the larynx was sacrificed. However, newer versions simultaneously provide a laryngoscopic and kymographic image simultaneously. The laryngoscopic image is used to select the position for capture of the kymographic image.[30,31] A digital kymograph generated from a patient with a vocal fold polyp is displayed in **Fig. 2**.

Unlike videostroboscopy in which many images are needed to analyze the vibrational pattern of the vocal folds, videokymography depicts the pattern in one image. The vibratory pattern may change along the length of the vocal fold, and therefore, multiple points may need to be evaluated. Videokymography has the potential to serve as an adjunct in the diagnosis of early glottic cancer. Schutte and colleagues[29] described the case of a patient who had previously undergone partial cordectomy and radiation therapy for laryngeal cancer who presented with persistent dysphonia. Vocal fold mobility was limited and stroboscopic evaluation revealed low-amplitude

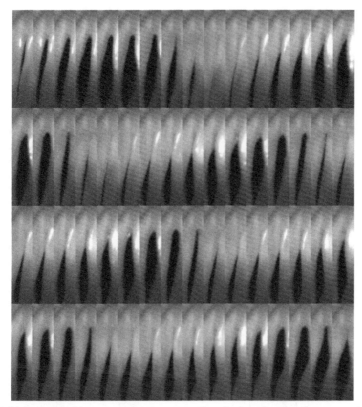

Fig. 1. A high-speed video montage demonstrating 5 glottal cycles from a patient with left vocal fold scar. There is asynchrony of cycle-to-cycle vibration. (Photo courtesy of Peak Woo, MD.)

vibration. Videokymography revealed no mucosal waves, suggesting tumor infiltration, which was later confirmed with biopsy.

OPTICAL COHERENCE TOMOGRAPHY

Optical coherence tomography (OCT) is an imaging technology that provides cross-sectional images of subsurface tissue structure at approximately 10-μm resolution to a depth of 1.2 mm using backscattered light. The tissue sample is probed with infrared light, and interferometric methods are used to detect light reflected from within the tissue.[32] Images are formed by dividing the light into 2 paths, one of which is directed at the tissue sample and another directed to a reference mirror. The light returning from the 2 paths is then compared. If the 2 paths have the same length and refractive index, the beams are identical or coherent and the signal will be above the threshold for detection. If the reference and probe beams have traveled different optical distances, the beams will not be coherent and there is destructive interference that prevents detection.[33] This interference results in selective detection of light from fixed depth within the tissue, which can be used to produce a 2-dimensional image. In the larynx, the image formed can provide information regarding the structure of the vocal folds that is analogous to a vertical histologic section.[34] Both benign and malignant vocal fold lesions may disrupt the mucosal layer of the vocal fold, leading to

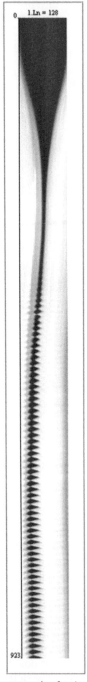

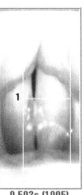

0.502s (1005)

Fig. 2. A digital kymograph of voice onset in a patient with a vocal fold polyp. The onset of vocal fold vibration that is delayed with reduced amplitude on the right. (Photo courtesy of Peak Woo, MD.)

dysphonia. OCT offers a noninvasive method to characterize the structure of the epithelium and SLP in both normal vocal folds and in pathologic conditions and may be a valuable tool in both diagnosis and treatment planning.

OCT has been shown to provide information regarding the thickness of the epithelium, integrity of the basement membrane, and the structure of the lamina propria.[35] Maturo and colleagues[36] showed that OCT may be used to quantitatively analyze the layers of the lamina propria of the vocal fold. This feature of OCT has the potential to help to characterize the subepithelial development of the pediatric vocal fold and help determine the need for operative intervention in children with dysphonia. OCT has also been shown to have utility in guiding subepithelial injections into the vocal folds in real-time.[37]

Polarization-sensitive optical coherence tomography (PS-OCT) is an additional form of OCT imaging that measures the intensity and polarization of state change of reflected light within the tissue in order to simultaneously characterize tissue structure and birefringence.[38] Collagen fibers are birefringent and can change the polarization state of reflected light; thus, PS-OCT can detect the collagen content of the vocal ligament that differs from the overlying SLP, which contains much less collagen.[34] Normal vocal fold tissue has a well-defined junction between the epithelium, which has low signal intensity, and the SLP, which has higher signal intensity and lacks significant structure, creating a light-dark-light banding pattern at the epithelium-SLP junction on PS-OCT images that indicates the presence of collagen in the SLP.[39]

The ability of OCT and PS-OCT to noninvasively provide information about vocal fold structure gives it the potential to be a valuable adjunct in the diagnosis of early glottic malignancies. OCT provides valuable information about the structure of the vocal folds in benign, premalignant, and malignant conditions. It has the potential to guide biopsies and treatment as well as monitor disease progression and response to therapy.[35] As previously described, PS-OCT and OCT can differentiate between the vocal ligament and SLP because of their differences in collagen content. This difference in tissue content allows these modalities to potentially identify epithelial lesions that disrupt the normal collagen pattern, such as invasive carcinoma.[34] Burns and colleagues[39] used PS-OCT and OCT to characterize the cross-sectional structure of the vocal folds of patients undergoing microlaryngoscopy for both benign and malignant lesions. Compared with normal glottic tissue, scar tissue displayed a more intense birefringence pattern, whereas cancer showed disruption or absence of the layered structure of the vocal fold and the birefringence pattern. In the vocal fold, biopsies and resections of lesions can lead to scarring that can have adverse effects on the voice of varying severity. PS-OCT and OCT could guide more accurate biopsies and resections by distinguishing potentially malignant areas from scar tissue or inflammation, thus preserving maximal normal tissue and improving functional outcomes.

AUTOFLUORESCENCE

Autofluorescence (AF) is the natural fluorescence emission of tissue arising from endogenous fluorophores after exposure and activation by radiation of a suitable wavelength. Its clinical utility stems from the fact that premalignant and malignant lesions can be differentiated from normal tissue because of decreased AF.[40] Autofluorescence endoscopy (AFE) has been applied in several medical specialties to detect malignant mucosal changes.[41–44] The different fluorescence emissions in AFE are due to neoplasia-induced changes in tissue morphology, optical properties, and the concentration of endogenous fluorophores.[45] The intracellular fluorophores, nicotinamide adenine dinucleotide plus hydrogen and flavin adenine dinucleotide, are found in all tissue layers, but their concentration is nearly 100 times lower in malignant tissue than in benign tissue.[46] Collagen and elastin are structural proteins and extracellular fluorophores that are found in subepithelial layers. Epithelial thickening of malignant and premalignant tissue also inhibits the penetration of exciting light into submucous layers, which also accounts for the reduced AF in neoplastic tissue.[47]

As described, the differences in AF properties of malignant and benign tissues make this technology extremely useful in the diagnosis of early glottic cancers. Several studies have demonstrated the utility of AF in the larynx. Harries and colleagues[48] in 1995 applied the lung imaging fluorescence endoscopy system, which uses a helium-cadmium laser light source (442-nm wavelength), to laryngeal lesions. By comparing biopsy specimens of areas of laryngeal mucosa with decreased AF (reddish-brown coloration) to specimens taken from mucosa with normal AF (green coloration), they established that this technology could effectively identify malignant lesions of the larynx. Zargi and colleagues[49] compared AF to standard white light microlaryngoscopy in 108 patients and found sensitivities of 86.9% and 71%, respectively, for identifying malignant lesions in the larynx. Specificities were 82.8% and 80.6%, respectively. Combining the 2 methods yielded a sensitivity of 97.1% for cancerous lesions and 61.5% for precancerous lesions, with an overall specificity of 71.8%. They determined that incorrect assessments were due to bleeding, which can cause a false positive impression of malignancy because surface blood can diminish AF of underlying tissue; hyperemia, due to increased presence of blood within the tissue; and leukoplakia, which emits strong AF and can result in a false negative assessment in some instances. False positives may also be due to mild dysplasia with inflammatory reactions or vocal fold scarring.[50] AF has also been applied through indirect laryngoscopy and shown to be a useful modality in the identification of early laryngeal cancers. Arens and colleagues[51] generated AF images via a 70° rigid-angled endoscope and found 89% concordance with histopathology resulted in the identification of laryngeal malignancy. AF has been applied during transoral laser resection of early laryngeal cancers. Succo and colleagues[52] performed a prospective cohort study with 73 patients undergoing CO_2 laser resection of early glottic cancers. The use of AF was associated with superficial disease-free margins in 97.2% of cases and superficial close margins in 2.8%. Diagnostic accuracy was improved in 16.4%, and 8.2% of cases were upstaged as a result of AF use. They reported a sensitivity of 96.5% and a specificity of 98.5%. They concluded that AF can help identify positive superficial margins intraoperatively, leading to improved local control and disease-specific survival.

When aminolevulinic acid (ALA) is applied topically to laryngeal mucosa, it preferentially induces fluorescence within neoplastic cells; this is due to its role in heme synthesis: 2 ALA molecules condense to form porphobilinogen, which is then metabolized to fluorophore protoporphyrin IX (PTP). The enzyme ferrochelatase incorporates Fe+ into PTP to form heme, which is not a fluorophore. Neoplastic cells are more permeable to ALA and thus accumulate PTP, whereas ferrochelatase production is downregulated.[53–55] Thus, when mucosa is treated with ALA, neoplastic cells emit the orange-red color of PTP, whereas healthy mucosa fluoresces green.[56] Several studies have compared ALA-induced fluorescence to AF and found similar accuracy between the 2 modalities in the diagnosis of laryngeal dysplasia and invasive carcinoma.[51,57,58] However, the addition of ALA-induced fluorescence to AF does not improve diagnostic accuracy.[59] ALA-induced fluorescence may also be better than AF in differentiating recurrent cancer from scar tissue after laser surgery.[51] Like AF, ALA-induced fluorescence cannot be used to determine histologic detail and thus cannot characterize grade of dysplasia or identify invasive carcinoma.

BIOLOGIC ENDOSCOPY TECHNIQUES
Contact Endoscopy and Confocal Endomicroscopy

Contact endoscopy (CE) is a technique that allows the surgeon to visualize cellular detail in vivo. A magnifying endoscope is placed in direct contact with the mucosa surface and delivers images at 60 or 150 times magnification.[60,61] Topical application of methylene blue to the mucosa stains nucleic acids and provides contrast between cell nuclei, which stain dark blue, and the lightly stained cytoplasm. Because of their higher mitotic rate, neoplastic cells stain more strongly.[62] Blood vessels also stain with methylene blue, which allows for the identification of angiogenesis.[61] These features allow histologic interpretations to be made in vivo and thus can aid in the identification of malignancy and identify disease margins. In addition to aiding in the identification of malignant cells, CE may also be used to characterize the degree of dysplasia of laryngeal lesions by identifying the degree of atypia within cells. Invasive carcinoma can also be reliably indicated by CE. Areas of invasion are characterized by tortuous vessels within the lamina propria deep to epithelium showing features of cellular atypia.[63] CE images, however, have been shown to be less sensitive than histologic analysis by frozen section in diagnosing invasive carcinoma when each modality is compared with analysis of paraffin-fixed tissue samples (78% and 100%, respectively).[64] A major limitation of CE is its inability to differentiate between CIS and invasive carcinoma of the larynx. CE cannot give clear images of cells beyond the superficial layers of the epithelium because, at high magnification, image resolution is significantly impacted by glare from light reflected by cells that are not in focus. Thus, CE cannot determine whether neoplastic cells breach the basement membrane.[56]

Confocal endomicroscopy (CEM) is an additional biologic endoscopy system that overcomes some of the shortcomings of CE. By eliminating out-of-focus light, CEM allows lesions to be examined in 3 dimensions, with magnification high enough to allow visualization beyond the basement membrane. An objective lens focuses a high-intensity illuminating light onto a small area of tissue, called the focal point. Light is then reflected back through the objective lens and focused on the confocal image detector. The detector is located behind a small pinhole, which filters light from outside the focal point and thus prevents it from reaching the detector. A high-resolution image of cells at the focal point is generated. The confocal microscope scans along the tissue at a single depth and captures images from numerous adjacent focal points in order to create a 2-dimensional image. The focal plane can be moved through the tissue to view cells at different depths, and by reviewing images at different focal planes, the tissue's 3-dimensional structure can be characterized. Thus, this modality has been referred to as a virtual biopsy.[65,66] With the addition of acriflavine hydrochloride (AH) stains, which stains cell nuclei, and intravenous administration of fluorescein, which attaches to serum albumin and thus highlights blood vessels, cellular and structural details of the tissue can be identified. Fluorescein also leaks through blood vessels to stain cell cytoplasm and the extracellular matrix.[67,68] With the administration of both AH and fluorescein, the sizes of cell nuclei can be compared with those of the surrounding cytoplasm. This comparison can help to identify cells near the basement membrane (smaller size, increased nucleus to cytoplasm ratio) and may help differentiate normal cells from CIS or invasive carcinoma.[67] CEM has been incorporated into flexible endoscopes and first applied to the imaging of the gastrointestinal tract.[69] With this system, 475-μm^2 images can be captured at 4-μm increments up to 250 μm from the mucosa surface in vivo. These 2-dimensional images are then projected onto a screen in real-time, allowing for intraoperative visualization of these sections.[67] A rigid endoscope equipped with CEM has also been developed, with improved sensitivity and handling in the larynx.[70] Although CEM is now well established in gastroenterology, its application to the diagnosis and treatment of laryngeal cancers is new and in the experimental stage. Given the risk of scarring and poor voice and swallowing outcomes due to biopsy and resection of glottic lesions, CEM is particularly applicable in the diagnosis and treatment of laryngeal neoplasms because of its ability to characterize cellular structure and guide more targeted biopsies as well as more precise margins of resection. Pogorzelski and colleagues[71] applied CEM via a rigid endoscope during endoscopy of 15 patients with SCC of the oral cavity, oropharynx, hypopharynx, or larynx. They were able to differentiate dysplastic and malignant mucosal changes from normal mucosa. They found good correlation between the CEM findings and histologic analysis of the tissue. Although not yet widely used, CEM offers promise in advancing the diagnosis and follow-up of glottic neoplasms and may be used with voice professionals where compromise of vocal quality from biopsy may be significantly detrimental to the patient's overall life.

Raman Spectroscopy

Raman spectroscopy (RS) is an additional noninvasive laryngeal imaging technique that can potentially identify tumors' molecular margins through analysis of a tissue's molecular composition. RS is based on the principle that intramolecular bonds cause light to scatter in a predictable and measurable way.[72] It is a noninvasive analysis of inelastic scattered photons following monochromatic laser excitation and provides information about the chemical and morphologic structure of tissue in real-time.[73] Most biological molecules, including proteins, nucleic acids, cell membranes, single cells, and tissues, are Raman active, have their own characteristic spectral fingerprint, and can be characterized with RS.[74] The monochromatic light source is usually near the infrared range to minimize the fluorescence background from tissue. The light collected from the tissue is then separated in its individual wavelengths through diffraction grating following filtration of the elastic scattered light at the laser wavelength. The Raman shift, which is the variation of each wavelength from the illuminating light, is calculated and plotted against intensity into a spectrum.[56]

RS, through its ability to analyze tissues' molecular structure, can help differentiate between benign and malignant tissue. Tissues have distinct spectral signatures determined by the biological molecules that comprise them. RS has previously been applied in in vitro studies to differentiate between pathologic abnormalities in several tissues including colon, esophagus, skin, bladder, and prostate gland.[56] Stone and colleagues[74] applied RS to biopsy specimens of laryngeal mucosa from 15 patients that were also examined histologically and classified as normal, dysplastic, or SCC. The Raman spectra of 7 samples of normal laryngeal mucosa were consistent between samples, and the normal spectra were compared with those of dysplastic and malignant tissue samples. They found a 90% specificity and 92% sensitivity for diagnosing invasive cancer using RS. In another in vitro study, Lau and colleagues[75] compared RS of 20 laryngeal samples recorded over a period of 5 seconds to histologic analysis of the same samples. RS showed a 94% specificity and 69% sensitivity for invasive carcinoma. Lin and colleagues[76] applied high wave number RS, which provides stronger tissue Raman signals with reduced tissue/fiber fluorescence background, in vivo to laryngeal mucosa via a flexible endoscope. With this type of RS as well, there are characteristic Raman spectra for benign and cancerous tissues. They compared the RS spectra with biopsy specimens and found a 90.9% specificity and 90.3% sensitivity for laryngeal cancer identification with high wave number RS via this system. Through its ability to differentiate malignant from benign tissue based on molecular composition, RS can potentially identify the true margins of laryngeal tumors.

Narrow Band Imaging

Narrow band imaging (NBI) is an optical technique that illuminates the intraepithelial papillary capillary loop using narrow bandwidth filters in a red-green-blue sequential illumination system.[77,78] In order to support their growth requirements, all kinds of tumors require the recruitment of surrounding blood vessels and vascular endothelial cells. Tumors promote the growth of new blood vessels from pre-existing ones, and these new vessels have characteristic features including chaotic blood flow, tortuous and dilated structure, and excessive branches and connections. Their walls have many openings, widened interendothelial junctions, and a discontinuous or absent basement membrane.[79] The NBI filter sets are 415 nm and 540 nm to provide images of the microvascular structure. Blue light, with a wavelength of 415 nm, is the hemoglobin absorption band, and therefore, capillaries on the surface of mucosa can be clearly visualized at this wavelength. The wavelength for green light is 540 nm, which penetrates the deeper tissues to enhance subepithelial vessels. **Fig. 3** shows an example of a laryngeal image generated with NBI compared with a stroboscopic image from the same patient. NBI displays capillary patterns and can identify boundaries between different types of tissues, which can aid in the early identification of tumors.[77,78] Superficial mucosal lesions that may be missed by white light endoscopy can be identified by their neoangiogenic pattern. In the head and neck, this technology has also been applied to the oropharynx, hypopharynx, and oral cavity. In these areas, superficial carcinoma appears as brown dots in a well-demarcated brownish area under NBI. This appearance is due to the microvascular proliferation pattern.[80–82] Piazza and colleagues[83] applied NBI coupled with a high-definition television camera both preoperatively and intraoperatively to 279 patients either undergoing workup for laryngeal SCC or who had previously undergone treatment of the condition. The findings obtained with NBI were compared with histologic analysis of biopsy samples, and high-definition NBI showed an overall sensitivity of 98% with a specificity of 90%. Kraft and colleagues[84] compared NBI to conventional white light endoscopy in patients with suspected laryngeal malignancies and compared the findings of each modality with biopsy results. They found sensitivities of 97% versus 79% for NBI and white light endoscopy, respectively. Accuracies were 97% versus 90%, respectively, and

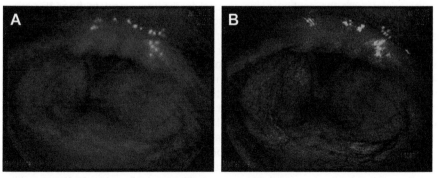

Fig. 3. (*A*) A stroboscopic photograph of a patient with posterior mucosal hypertrophy. (*B*) NBI photograph of the same patient, highlighting the surface vasculature of the larynx.

specificities were 96% and 95%, respectively. Ni and colleagues[85] described a classification system for vascular patterns observed in the larynx using NBI. They designated 5 types (I–V) based on the vascular features of the intraepithelial papillary capillary loop, with types I–IV corresponding to nonmalignant lesions and type V being malignant. They found that this classification correlated well with the histologic examinations of the laryngeal lesions they studied. Bertino and colleagues[86] applied NBI using the Ni classification to 248 patients with pharyngolaryngeal lesions and found sensitivity, specificity, accuracy, positive predictive value (PPV), and negative predictive value (NPV) of 97.4%, 84.6%, 92.7%, 91.6%, and 95.1%, respectively. Ninety-eight percent of malignant lesions by histologic examination corresponded to a type V NBI pattern, and 84.8% of benign lesions corresponded to a type I–IV pattern. NBI has also been applied more specifically to the follow-up of patients treated for laryngeal and hypopharyngeal carcinoma, conditions in which early detection of recurrent disease is often difficult. Zabrodsky and colleagues[87] applied NBI via transnasal flexible videoendoscopy in an ambulatory setting to 66 patients previously treated for laryngeal or hypopharyngeal cancer with radiation or chemotherapy. Suspicious lesions identified by NBI were then biopsied, and they found an accuracy of 88%, sensitivity of 92%, specificity of 76%, PPV of 96%, and a NPV of 91%. The investigators also asserted that many of the lesions identified were not seen with white light endoscopy. In addition to aiding in the diagnosis and treatment of laryngeal malignancies, NBI has also been shown to be a useful adjunct in the management of recurrent respiratory papillomatosis.[88,89]

COMPUTED TOMOGRAPHY, MRI, PET, AND ULTRASOUND

Accurate determination of the disease stage is essential to delineating treatment options and choosing the best therapeutic strategy for the patient. Diagnostic imaging modalities are helpful in the clinical staging of glottic malignancies and can determine if there is involvement of deep structures, such as the anterior commissure, thyroid cartilage, or paraglottic space, and identify any suspicious nodal enlargement.

Computed Tomography

Computed tomography (CT) can identify tumors in the larynx as well as other head and neck subsites based on either anatomic distortion or tumor enhancement. On CT, tumors enhance more than normal head and neck structures with the exception of mucosa, blood vessels, and extraocular muscles.[90] Standard CT imaging for laryngeal cancer is contrast-enhanced helical CT scan from the C1 vertebral body to the thoracic inlet, with the section plane parallel to the true vocal folds or the hyoid bone, with the section thickness not exceeding 3 mm.[91] Compared with MRI, CT offers greater spatial resolution and is performed with faster acquisition times, nearly eliminating motion artifact. CT is also better than MRI for the evaluation of bony anatomy. CT scans performed for laryngeal pathologic abnormality should be reconstructed using soft tissue algorithms, with a high-resolution bone algorithm in the area extending from the thyroid cartilage to the base of the cricoid cartilage to evaluate for cartilage invasion by tumor. Through the evaluation of sclerosis, erosion, lysis, and extralaryngeal spread, CT imaging of the larynx can achieve a 91% sensitivity and 95% NPV for the detection of cartilage invasion.[91]

CT scan can also provide information about regional lymph node involvement. CT evaluation relies on size criteria to differentiate involved from uninvolved lymph nodes and can also detect extracapsular spread. Radiographically, pathologic lymphadenopathy is defined as a node measuring greater than 10 to 11 mm in minimal axial diameter or one that contains central necrosis.[92,93] Other features that suggest a pathologic lymph node include rounded shape, loss of fatty hilum, and increased or heterogeneous contrast enhancement. CT has been shown to be superior to physical examination in detecting pathologic lymphadenopathy. One meta-analysis of studies comparing CT scan with physical examination found an overall sensitivity of 83% versus 74%, respectively, specificity of 83% versus 81%, respectively, accuracy of 83% versus 77%, respectively, and detection of cervical lymphadenopathy of 91% versus 75%, respectively.[94] CT scan does have limitations in the detection of nodal metastases related to size criteria. In a study of 957 cervical lymph nodes from patients with head and neck cancer, 102 (11%) contained malignant cells. Of those, 67% were 10 mm or smaller and thus would not have been identified as potentially pathologic on CT scan.[95] Lymphatic spread in early glottic cancer, however, is rare.

MRI

MRI offers some advantages over CT in the evaluation of glottic malignancy, including greater soft tissue definition.[96] With respect to the primary tumor, MRI may be more helpful in identifying disease involvement of the laryngeal ventricle and transglottic spread on coronal imaging. Midsagittal MRI can characterize the involvement of the anterior commissure. One disadvantage of MRI, however, is the longer imaging time, which may result in poorer image quality due to motion artifact. MRI of the larynx can reveal cartilage involvement, with hypointensity on T1-weighted images, hyperintensity on T2-weighted images, and gadolinium enhancement signifying the possibility of cartilage invasion by tumor. Involvement of the overlying strap muscle, however, is the only truly diagnostic indicator of cartilage invasion on MRI. The sensitivity of MRI in predicting cartilage invasion has been reported as 89% to 94%, with a specificity of 74% to 88% and an NPV of 94% to 96%.[91] Allegra and colleagues[97] reported MRI and CT findings in patients with early glottic cancers and compared the 2 modalities with the final pathology reports after biopsy. CT showed a diagnostic accuracy of 70% compared with 80% for MRI. MRI showed a sensitivity of 100% and a specificity of 97% in assessing the paraglottic space, anterior commissure, thyroid, and arytenoid cartilages. CT showed a specificity of 100% but a sensitivity of 40%. The investigators concluded that MRI may be a superior study to CT for evaluation of early glottic neoplasms and treatment planning, especially determining the appropriateness of conservative surgery.

MRI has been shown to be inferior to CT scan in the detection of cervical adenopathy, with sensitivities reported to be as low as 57% to 67%. New contrast agents are emerging that show promise in improving the ability of MRI to detect nodal metastases. Dextran-coated ultrasmall supramagnetic iron oxide (USPIO) is a substance that is administered intravenously and is taken up by macrophages in lymph nodes. The signal intensity of normal lymph nodes on T1 and T2 MRI sequences after administration of USPIO is markedly reduced because of uptake of the iron particles by macrophages. Metastatic lymph nodes do not lose signal on contrast-enhanced images because the macrophages have been replaced. The sensitivity and specificity of detecting nodal metastases using USPIO have been reported as 87% and 90%, respectively.[98]

PET

Although PET is not routinely used in the evaluation and treatment planning of early glottic neoplasms, its role is highlighted in the staging of more advanced glottic cancers and monitoring after treatment. PET imaging is based on the increased glycolytic activity of neoplastic cells. Injected positron-emitting radionuclides, such as fluorine-18, are taken up by metabolically or functionally active tissues. The emissions are detected and reconstructed to produce a 3-dimensional image. The most common agent used is 18F-fluorodeoxyglucose (FDG), which is taken up by cells in different concentrations depending on the metabolism of the tissue. Metabolic rates are high in most tumors, leading to increased update and detection by PET. PET itself has poor spatial resolution and alone is limited in its ability to localize primary tumor site and regional lymph node metastases in the head and neck. Lowe and colleagues,[99] however, found that FDG-PET was able to detect primary or recurrent early-stage laryngeal tumors in 11 of 12 patients with biopsy-proven tumors. Nine of the patients had undergone CT scan that was read as normal in 6 cases. Combining PET with CT scan improves anatomic localization, and the 2 studies can be performed sequentially on a hybrid PET/CT scanner. The images are the fused allowing anatomic localization of the PET signals. PET/CT is still limited by its inability to detect small tumors less than 3 to 4 mm, but this may improve as the technology advances. In patients with known early-stage laryngeal malignancy, some advocate baseline PET/CT for comparison at posttreatment follow-up.[100] In one meta-analysis, PET scan alone showed an 89% specificity and a specificity of 74% for detecting recurrent laryngeal cancer after treatment.[101]

As far as the ability of PET to detect nodal metastases in laryngeal cancer, most data have shown PET to be more useful in detecting nodal disease in higher T-stage tumors, where the lymph nodes are more likely to be involved. One meta-analysis showed an overall 79% sensitivity of PET for detecting cervical lymph node metastases, but this dropped to 50% in clinically N0 nodes.[102] Another study found a 100% detection rate when the short axis of the metastatic lymph node was greater than or equal to 1 cm. No involved lymph nodes less than 5 mm were detected.[103] Based on these findings, PET scan has limited application in the initial workup of early glottic malignancies in which nodal metastases are rare.

Ultrasound

Ultrasound (US) imaging has recently been applied to the workup of disorders of the larynx, including carcinoma. US is routinely used for the detection of cervical lymph node metastases in head and neck cancer as well as to assess thyroid gland involvement in advanced laryngeal tumors, but has not been widely applied to the staging of primary laryngeal malignancies. Color Doppler US has been used to noninvasively assess mucosal wave velocity and the elasticity of the vocal folds. The pseudocolor codes of the US image were used to infer the vocal fold displacement velocity, providing information about phonatory function in disorders that affect vocal fold vibration.[104] Unlike CT and MRI, US has the ability to detect and characterize vocal fold motion. Hu and colleagues[105] used high-frequency US to stage 36 laryngeal tumors, 21 of which arose from the glottis. The findings on US and CT scan were then compared with final pathologic analysis of the tumor after resection to determine accuracy. They found a T-staging accuracy of 83.3% compared with 88.8% for CT. There was not a statistically significant difference between the 2 modalities except in the evaluation of tumor involvement of retrolaryngeal structures, in which CT scan was superior. A study by Xia and colleagues[106] comparing high-frequency US to CT for the staging of laryngeal cancer found US to have a lower rate of detection of laryngeal cancers than CT (87.5% vs 100%). Sensitivity and specificity were similar for the 2 modalities, except US was more specific for identifying tumor involvement of the paraglottic space (94.9% vs 66.7% for CT).

An additional application of US to laryngeal cancer is through endosonography, in which a US probe is used to evaluate endolaryngeal structure during direct laryngoscopy. The probes have penetrating depths of 10 to 25 mm and a high tissue resolution.[107] Endosonography produces horizontal slice images comparable to CT or MRI but with higher resolution. Kraft and colleagues[108] compared endosonography of laryngeal tumors with CT and MRI and found that endosonography had the highest accuracy for the staging of laryngeal cancer (89% vs 77% for both CT and MRI). Although this technology has not been widely applied, it offers promise as a modality for determining the depth of tumor and involvement of adjacent structures during direct laryngoscopy and could be a valuable staging tool for laryngeal carcinoma.

SUMMARY

Laryngeal cancer is a disease that may result in significant morbidity and mortality, especially if diagnosis and treatment are delayed. Identifying potentially malignant lesions early and initiating the appropriate treatment results in improved outcomes. Imaging of the larynx is integral to early diagnosis of glottic neoplasms and to follow-up after treatment. Significant advances continue to be made in the ability to visualize the larynx, and it is hoped that these will continue to improve outcomes in patients with glottic malignancies as their availability increases.

REFERENCES

1. Parkin DM, Bray F, Ferlay J, et al. Global cancer statistics, 2002. CA Cancer J Clin 2005;55:74–108.
2. American Joint Committee on Cancer. American Cancer Society, American College of Surgeons. AJCC Staging Manual. 6th edition. Philadelphia: Lippincott-Raven; 2002. p. 47–57.
3. Marioni G, Marchese-Ragona R, Cartei G, et al. Current opinion in diagnosis and treatment of laryngeal carcinoma. Cancer Treat Rev 2006;32:504–15.
4. Hoffman HT, Porter K, Karnell LH, et al. Laryngeal cancer in the United States: changes in demographics, patterns of care, and survival. Laryngoscope 2006; 116(9 Pt 2 Suppl 111):1–13.
5. Ferlito A. The natural history of early vocal cord cancer. Acta Otolaryngol 1995; 115(2):345–7.
6. Huang BY, Solle M, Weissler MC. Larynx: anatomic imaging for diagnosis and management. Otolaryngol Clin North Am 2012;45(6):1325–61.
7. Batsakis JG. Surgical excision margins: a pathologist's perspective. Adv Anat Pathol 1999;6:140–8.
8. Isenberg JS, Crozier DL, Dailey SH. Institutional and comprehensive review of laryngeal leukoplakia. Ann Otol Rhinol Laryngol 2008;117(1):74–9.
9. Popolo PS, Titze IR. Qualification of a quantitative laryngeal imaging system using videostroboscopy and videokymography. Ann Otol Rhinol Laryngol 2008; 117:404–12.
10. Sulica L. Hoarseness. Arch Otolaryngol Head Neck Surg 2011;137:616–9.
11. Schwartz SR, Cohen SM, Dailey SH, et al. Clinical practice guideline: hoarseness (dysphonia). Otolaryngol Head Neck Surg 2009;141:S1–31.
12. Verikas A, Uloza V, Bacauskiene M, et al. Advances in laryngeal imaging. Eur Arch Otorhinolaryngol 2009;266(10):1509–20.
13. Rihkanen H, Reijonen P, Lehikoinen-Soderlund S, et al. Videostroboscopic assessment of unilateral vocal fold paralysis after augmentation with autologous fascia. Eur Arch Otorhinolaryngol 2004;261:177–83.
14. Sung MW, Kim KH, Koh TY, et al. Videostrobokymography: a new method for the quantitative analysis of vocal fold vibration. Laryngoscope 1999;109:1859–63.

15. Sulter AM, Schutte HK, Miller DG. Standardized laryngeal videostroboscopic rating: differences between untrained and trained male and female subjects, and effects of varying sound intensity fundamental frequency, and age. J Voice 1996;10:175–89.

16. Rosen CA, Gartner-Schmidt J, Hathaway B, et al. A nomenclature paradigm for benign midmembranous vocal fold lesions. Laryngoscope 2012;122: 1335–41.

17. Zhao R, Hirano M, Tanaka S, et al. Vocal fold epithelial hyperplasia: vibratory behavior versus extent of lesion. Arch Otolaryngol Head Neck Surg 1991;117: 1015–8.

18. Colden D, Zeitels SM, Hillman RE, et al. Stroboscopic assessment of vocal fold keratosis and glottic cancer. Ann Otol Rhinol Laryngol 2001;110:293–8.

19. Woo P. Objective measures of laryngeal imaging: what we have learned since Dr. Paul Moore. J Voice 2014;28(1):69–81.

20. Kitzing P. Stroboscopy—a pertinent laryngological examination. J Otolaryngol 1985;14:151–7.

21. Patel R, Dailey S, Bless D. Comparison of high-speed digital imaging with stroboscopy for laryngeal imaging of glottal disorders. Ann Otol Rhinol Laryngol 2008;117(6):413–24.

22. Jiang JJ, Yumoto E, Lin SJ, et al. Quantitative measurement of mucosal wave by high-speed photography in excised larynges. Ann Otol Rhinol Laryngol 1998; 107(2):98–103.

23. Mortensen M, Woo P. High-speed imaging used to detect vocal fold paresis: a case report. Ann Otol Rhinol Laryngol 2008;117:684–7.

24. Mendelsohn AH, Remacle M, Courey MS, et al. The diagnostic role of high-speed vocal fold vibratory imaging. J Voice 2013;27(5):627–31.

25. Bonilha HS, Deliyski DD. Period and glottal width irregularities in vocally normal speakers. J Voice 2008;22(6):699–708.

26. Bonilha HS, Deliyski DD, Gerlach TT. Phase asymmetries in normophonic speakers: visual judgments and objective findings. Am J Speech Lang Pathol 2008;17(4):367–76.

27. Krausert CR, Olszewski AE, Taylor LN, et al. Mucosal wave measurement and visualization techniques. J Voice 2011;25(4):395–405.

28. Svec JG, Schutte HK. Videokymography: high-speed line scanning of vocal fold vibration. J Voice 1996;10:201–5.

29. Schutte HK, Svec JG, Sram F. First results of clinical application of videokymography. Laryngoscope 1998;108:1206–10.

30. Qiu QJ, Schutte HK. A new generation videokymography for routine clinical vocal fold examination. Laryngoscope 2006;116:1824–8.

31. Qiu QJ, Schutte HK. Real-time kymographic imaging for visualizing human vocal-fold vibratory function. Rev Sci Instrum 2007;78:1–6.

32. Huang D, Swanson EA, Lin CP, et al. Optical coherence tomography. Science 1991;254:1178–83.

33. Podoleanu AG. Optical coherence tomography. Br J Radiol 2005;78:976–88.

34. Burns JA. Optical coherence tomography: imaging the larynx. Curr Opin Otolaryngol Head Neck Surg 2012;20(6):477–81.

35. Wong BJ, Jackson RP, Guo S, et al. In vivo optical coherence tomography of the human larynx: normative and benign pathology in 82 patients. Laryngoscope 2005;115(11):1904–11.

36. Maturo S, Benboujja F, Boudoux C, et al. Quantitative distinction of unique vocal fold subepithelial architectures. Ann Otol Rhinol Laryngol 2012;121(11):754–60.

37. Burns JA, Kim KH, Kobler JB, et al. Real-time tracking of vocal fold injections with optical coherence tomography. Laryngoscope 2009;119(11):2182–6.
38. deBoer JF, Milner TE. Review of polarization sensitive optical coherence tomography and stokes vector determination. J Biomed Opt 2002;7:359–71.
39. Burns JA, Kim KH, deBoer JF, et al. Polarization-sensitive optical coherence tomography imaging of benign and malignant laryngeal lesions: an in vivo study. Otolaryngol Head Neck Surg 2011;145(1):91–9.
40. Caffier PP, Schmidt B, Gross M, et al. A comparison of white light laryngostroboscopy versus autofluorescence endoscopy in the evaluation of vocal fold pathology. Laryngoscope 2013;123(7):1729–34.
41. Chen W, Gao X, Tian Q, et al. A comparison of autofluorescence bronchoscopy and white light bronchoscopy in detection of lung cancer and preneoplastic lesions: a meta-analysis. Lung Cancer 2011;73:183–8.
42. Jacobson MC, deVere White R, Demos SG. In vivo testing of a prototype system providing simultaneous white light and near infrared autofluorescence image acquisition for detection of bladder cancer. J Biomed Opt 2012;17:036011.
43. McAlpine JN, El Hallani S, Lam SF, et al. Autofluorescence imaging can identify preinvasive or clinically occult lesions in fallopian tube epithelium: a promising step towards screening and early detection. Gynecol Oncol 2011;120:385–92.
44. Sieron-Stoltny K, Kwiatek S, Latos W, et al. Autofluorescence endoscopy with "real-time" digital image processing in differential diagnostics of selected benign and malignant lesions in the oesophagus. Photodiagnosis Photodyn Ther 2012;9:5–10.
45. Wagnieres GA, Star WM, Wilson BC. In vivo fluorescence spectroscopy and imaging for oncological applications. Photochem Photobiol 1998;68:603–32.
46. Uppal A, Gupta PK. Measurement of NADH concentration in normal and malignant human tissues from breast and oral cavity. Biotechnol Appl Biochem 2003; 37(Pt 1):45–50.
47. Arens C, Glanz H, Wonckhaus J, et al. Histologic assessment of epithelial thickness in early laryngeal cancer or precursor lesions and its impact on endoscopic imaging. Eur Arch Otorhinolaryngol 2007;264:645–9.
48. Harries ML, Lam S, MacAulay C, et al. Diagnostic imaging of the larynx: autofluorescence of laryngeal tumours using the helium-cadmium laser. J Laryngol Otol 1995;109(2):108–10.
49. Zargi M, Fajdiga I, Smid L. Autofluorescence imaging in the diagnosis of laryngeal cancer. Eur Arch Otorhinolaryngol 2000;257(1):17–23.
50. Malzahn K, Dreyer T, Glanz H, et al. Autofluorescence endoscopy in the diagnosis of early laryngeal cancer and its precursor lesions. Laryngoscope 2002; 112(3):488–93.
51. Arens C, Dreyer T, Glanz H, et al. Indirect autofluorescence laryngoscopy in the diagnosis of laryngeal cancer and its precursor lesions. Eur Arch Otorhinolaryngol 2004;261(2):71–6.
52. Succo G, Garofalo P, Fantini M, et al. Direct autofluorescence during CO2 laser surgery of the larynx: can it really help the surgeon? Acta Otorhinolaryngol Ital 2014;34(3):174–83.
53. Abels C, Fritsch C, Bolsen K, et al. Photodynamic therapy with 5-aminolaevulinic acid-induced porphyrins of an amelanotic melanoma in vivo. J Photochem Photobiol B 1997;40:76–83.
54. Kennedy JC, Pottier RH. Endogenous protoporphyrin IX, a clinically useful photosensitizer for photodynamic therapy. J Photochem Photobiol B 1992;14: 275–92.

55. Kemmner W, Wan K, Ruttinger S, et al. Silencing of human ferrochelatase causes abundant protoporphyrin-IX accumulation in colon cancer. FASEB J 2008;22:500–9.

56. Hughes OR, Stone N, Kraft M, et al. Optical and molecular techniques to identify tumor margins within the larynx. Head Neck 2010;32(11):1544–53.

57. Mehlmann M, Betz CS, Stepp H, et al. Fluorescence staining of laryngeal neoplasms after topical application of 5-aminolevulinic acid: preliminary results. Lasers Surg Med 1999;25:414–20.

58. Csanady M, Kiss JG, Ivan L, et al. ALA (5-aminolevulinic acid)-induced protoporphyrin IX fluorescence in the endoscopic diagnostic and control of pharyngo-laryngeal cancer. Eur Arch Otorhinolaryngol 2004;261:262–6.

59. Rydell R, Eker C, Andersson-Engels S, et al. Fluorescence investigations to classify malignant laryngeal lesions in vivo. Head Neck 2008;30:419–26.

60. Andrea M, Dias O, Santos A. Contact endoscopy during microlaryngeal surgery: a new technique for endoscopic examination of the larynx. Ann Otol Rhinol Laryngol 1995;104:333–9.

61. Carriero E, Galli J, Fadda G, et al. Preliminary experiences with contact endoscopy of the larynx. Eur Arch Otorhinolaryngol 2000;257:68–71.

62. Chen YW, Lin JS, Wu CH, et al. Application of in vivo stain of methylene blue as a diagnostic aid in the early detection and screening of oral squamous cell carcinoma and precancer lesions. J Chin Med Assoc 2007;70:497–503.

63. Wardrop PJ, Sim S, McLaren K. Contact endoscopy of the larynx: a quantitative study. J Laryngol Otol 2000;114:437–40.

64. Cikojevic D, Gluncic I, Pesutic-Pisac V. Comparison of contact endoscopy and frozen section histopathology in the intraoperative diagnosis of laryngeal pathology. J Laryngol Otol 2008;122:836–9.

65. Amos W, White J. How the confocal laser scanning microscope entered biological research. Biol Cell 2003;95:335–42.

66. Kiesslich R, Burg J, Vieth M, et al. Confocal laser endoscopy for diagnosing intraepithelial neoplasias and colorectal cancer in vivo. Gastroenterology 2004; 127(3):706–13.

67. Hurlstone DP, Baraza W, Brown S, et al. In vivo real-time confocal laser scanning endomicroscopic colonoscopy for the detection and characterization of colorectal neoplasia. Br J Surg 2008;95:636–45.

68. Birchall M, Hurlstone D. Confocal endomicroscopy. Sheffield (United Kingdom): University of Sheffield; 2007.

69. Polglase AL, McLaren WJ, Skinner SA, et al. A fluorescence confocal endomicroscope for in vivo microscopy of the upper- and the lower-GI tract. Gastrointest Endosc 2005;62(5):686–95.

70. Just T, Pau HW. Intra-operative application of confocal endomicroscopy using a rigid endoscope. J Laryngol Otol 2013;127(6):599–604.

71. Pogorzelski B, Hanenkamp U, Goetz M, et al. Systematic intraoperative application of confocal endomicroscopy for early detection and resection of squamous cell carcinoma of the head and neck: a preliminary report. Arch Otolaryngol Head Neck Surg 2012;138(4):404–11.

72. Raman C, Krishnan K. A new type of secondary radiation. Nature 1928;121:501–2.

73. Barr H, Dix T, Stone N. Optical spectroscopy for the early diagnosis of gastrointestinal malignancy. Lasers Med Sci 1998;13:3–13.

74. Stone N, Stavroulaki P, Kendall C, et al. Raman spectroscopy for early detection of laryngeal malignancy: preliminary results. Laryngoscope 2000;110(10 Pt 1): 1756–63.

75. Lau DP, Huang Z, Lui H, et al. Raman spectroscopy for optical diagnosis in the larynx: preliminary findings. Lasers Surg Med 2005;37(3):192–200.

76. Lin K, Cheng DL, Huang Z. Optical diagnosis of laryngeal cancer using high wavenumber Raman spectroscopy. Biosens Bioelectron 2012;35(1):213–7.

77. Gono K, Yamazaki K, Doguchi N, et al. Endoscopic observation of tissue by narrow band illumination. Opt Rev 2003;10:211–5.

78. Gono K, Obi T, Yamaguchi M, et al. Appearance of enhanced tissue feature in narrow-band endoscopic imaging. J Biomed Opt 2004;9:568–77.

79. Carmeliet P, Jain RK. Angiogenesis in cancer and in other diseases. Nature 2000;407:249–57.

80. Muto M, Nakane M, Katada C, et al. Squamous cell carcinoma in situ at oropharyngeal and hypopharyngeal mucosal sites. Cancer 2004;101:1375–81.

81. Katada C, Nakayama M, Tanabe S, et al. Narrow band imaging for detecting superficial oral squamous cell carcinoma: a report of two cases. Laryngoscope 2007;117:1596–9.

82. Katada C, Nakayama M, Tanabe S, et al. Narrow band imaging for detecting metachronous superficial oropharyngeal and hypopharyngeal squamous cell carcinomas after chemoradiotherapy for head and neck cancers. Laryngoscope 2008;118:1787–90.

83. Piazza C, Cocco D, De Benedetto L, et al. Narrow band imaging and high definition television in the assessment of laryngeal cancer: a prospective study on 279 patients. Eur Arch Otorhinolaryngol 2010;267(3):409–14.

84. Kraft M, Fostiropoulos K, Gürtler N, et al. Value of narrow band imaging in the early diagnosis of laryngeal cancer. Head Neck 2014. [Epub ahead of print].

85. Ni XG, He S, Xu ZG, et al. Endoscopic diagnosis of laryngeal cancer and precancerous lesions by narrow band imaging. J Laryngol Otol 2011;125(3):288–96.

86. Bertino G, Cacciola S, Fernandes WB Jr, et al. Effectiveness of narrow band imaging in the detection of premalignant and malignant lesions of the larynx: validation of a new endoscopic clinical classification. Head Neck 2015;37(2):215–22.

87. Zabrodsky M, Lukes P, Lukesova E, et al. The role of narrow band imaging in the detection of recurrent laryngeal and hypopharyngeal cancer after curative radiotherapy. Biomed Res Int 2014;2014:175398.

88. Tjon Pian Gi RE, Halmos GB, van Hemel BM, et al. Narrow band imaging is a new technique in visualization of recurrent respiratory papillomatosis. Laryngoscope 2012;122(8):1826–30.

89. Imaizumi M, Okano W, Tada Y, et al. Surgical treatment of laryngeal papillomatosis using narrow band imaging. Otolaryngol Head Neck Surg 2012;147(3):522–4.

90. Weissman JL, Akindele R. Current imaging techniques for head and neck tumors. Oncology (Williston Park) 1999;13:697.

91. Becker M, Burkhardt K, Dulguerov P, et al. Imaging of the larynx and hypopharynx. Eur J Radiol 2008;66(3):460–79.

92. Anzai Y, Brunberg JA, Lufkin RB. Imaging of nodal metastases in the head and neck. J Magn Reson Imaging 1997;7:774.

93. Curtin HD, Ishwaran H, Mancuso AA, et al. Comparison of CT and MR imaging in staging of neck metastases. Radiology 1998;207:123.

94. Merritt RM, Williams MF, James TH, et al. Detection of cervical metastasis. A meta-analysis comparing computed tomography with physical examination. Arch Otolaryngol Head Neck Surg 1997;123:149.

95. Don DM, Anzai Y, Lufkin RB, et al. Evaluation of cervical lymph node metastases in squamous cell carcinoma of the head and neck. Laryngoscope 1995;105: 669.

96. Sakata K, Hareyama M, Tamakawa M, et al. Prognostic factors of nasopharynx tumors investigated by MR imaging and the value of MR imaging in the newly published TNM staging. Int J Radiat Oncol Biol Phys 1999;43:273.

97. Allegra E, Ferrise P, Trapasso S, et al. Early glottic cancer: role of MRI in the pre-operative staging. Biomed Res Int 2014;2014:890385.

98. Sadick M, Schoenberg SO, Hoermann K, et al. Current oncologic concepts and emerging techniques for imaging of head and neck squamous cell cancer. GMS Curr Top Otorhinolaryngol Head Neck Surg 2012;11:Doc08.

99. Lowe VJ, Kim H, Boyd JH, et al. Primary and recurrent early stage laryngeal cancer: preliminary results of 2-[fluorine 18]fluoro-2-deoxy-D-glucose PET imaging. Radiology 1999;212(3):799–802.

100. Chu MM, Kositwattanarerk A, Lee DJ, et al. FDG PET with contrast-enhanced CT: a critical imaging tool for laryngeal carcinoma. Radiographics 2010;30(5): 1353–72.

101. Brouwer J, Hooft L, Hoekstra OS, et al. Systematic review: accuracy of imaging tests in the diagnosis of recurrent laryngeal carcinoma after radiotherapy. Head Neck 2008;30(7):889–97.

102. Kyzas PA, Evangelou E, Denaxa-Kyza D, et al. 18F-fluorodeoxyglucose positron emission tomography to evaluate cervical node metastases in patients with head and neck squamous cell carcinoma: a meta-analysis. J Natl Cancer Inst 2008;100(10):712–20.

103. Yamazaki Y, Saitoh M, Notani K, et al. Assessment of cervical lymph node metastases using FDG-PET in patients with head and neck cancer. Ann Nucl Med 2008;22(3):177–84.

104. Shau YW, Wang CL, Hsieh FJ, et al. Noninvasive assessment of vocal fold mucosal wave velocity using color doppler imaging. Ultrasound Med Biol 2001;27(11):1451–60.

105. Hu Q, Luo F, Zhu SY, et al. Staging of laryngeal carcinoma: comparison of high-frequency sonography and contrast-enhanced computed tomography. Clin Radiol 2012;67(2):140–7.

106. Xia CX, Zhu Q, Zhao HX, et al. Usefulness of ultrasonography in assessment of laryngeal carcinoma. Br J Radiol 2013;86(1030):20130343.

107. Kraft M, Arens C. Technique of high-frequency endolaryngeal ultrasound. J Laryngol Otol 2008;122(10):1109–11.

108. Kraft M, Bruns N, Hügens-Penzel M, et al. Clinical value of endosonography in the assessment of laryngeal cancer. Head Neck 2013;35(2):195–200.

Preserving Voice in Early Laryngeal Cancer

Laryngeal Function After Radiation Therapy

Mauricio Gamez, MD[a], Kenneth Hu, MD[b], Louis B. Harrison, MD[c],*

KEYWORDS

- Function • Speech • Voice • Dysphagia

KEY POINTS

- Radiation therapy is one of the treatments of choice for patients with larynx cancer with the goal of organ and function preservation.
- The oncologic and functional outcomes with radiation therapy are good.
- We review the subject in comprehensive detail.

INTRODUCTION

Head and neck cancer (HNC) accounts for more than 550,000 cases annually worldwide.[1] Males are affected significantly more than females with a ratio of 2:1 to 4:1. In the United States, HNC accounts for 3% of all malignancies, with an estimated 55,000 Americans developing HNC annually and 12,000 dying from the disease.[2] The incidence of laryngeal cancer in the United States is approximately 12,000 cases per year representing around 20% of all HNC with more than 95% being squamous cell carcinoma.

In early stage glottic larynx cancer, the standard treatment options are radiation therapy (RT) or partial laryngectomy/cordectomy (CO_2 laser). Although partial laryngectomy or cordectomy produces comparable cure rates for selected T1 and T2 vocal cord lesions, RT is generally preferred in most centers because of a better voice quality after treatment.[3]

Until the early 1990s, the standard treatment of locally advanced laryngeal squamous cell carcinoma unsuitable for function-preservation surgery was total laryngectomy and adjuvant RT. Although this approach is effective and produces high rates

Disclosures: None.
[a] Department of Radiation Oncology, Mayo Clinic Hospital, Mayo Clinic Arizona, Mayo Clinic Specialty Building, 5777 East Mayo Boulevard, Phoenix, AZ 85054, USA; [b] Department of Radiation Oncology, NYU-Langone Medical Center, 550 First avenue, New York, NY 10016, USA; [c] Department of Radiation Oncology, Moffitt Cancer Center, 12902 Magnolia Drive, Tampa, FL 33612, USA
* Corresponding author.
E-mail address: Louis.harrison@moffitt.org

Otolaryngol Clin N Am 48 (2015) 585–599
http://dx.doi.org/10.1016/j.otc.2015.04.005
0030-6665/15/$ – see front matter © 2015 Elsevier Inc. All rights reserved.

of local control, it results in a permanent tracheostomy. This can have a negative impact on patient function and quality of life, with such consequences as depression and social isolation.[4] More recently, different treatment strategies using RT alone, induction chemotherapy, or concurrent chemoradiotherapy (CRT) have been developed with the goal to preserve laryngeal function without compromising locoregional control and ultimate survival.[5–8]

Pfister and colleagues[8] reported one of the first series of larynx preservation with combined chemotherapy and RT. They included 40 patients with advanced, resectable squamous cell carcinoma of the larynx, oropharynx, and hypopharynx whose surgery would have required total laryngectomy. Patients were treated with one to three cycles of induction cisplatin-based chemotherapy before local therapy. Thirty-one of 40 patients (78%) had no evidence of disease at a median follow-up of 49 months. The overall survival was 58% at 2 years and 33% at 5 years. The actual larynx-preservation rate was 85% suggesting that this multidisciplinary treatment approach was feasible and effective.

Other trials had reported their larynx-preservation outcomes with the use of induction chemotherapy or CRT. The Veterans Affairs Laryngeal Cancer Study Group trial randomized patients to total laryngectomy followed by postoperative radiation versus induction CRT, showing a 2-year larynx-preservation rate of 64%.[5] Subsequently, the Radiation Therapy Oncology Group 91–11 established concurrent CRT as an effective strategy for organ preservation in advanced laryngeal squamous cell carcinoma. This trial randomized patients to combined CRT versus induction chemotherapy versus RT alone. The rates of laryngeal preservation at 3.8 years were 84%, 72%, and 67%, respectively, in favor of the combined modality arm.[6] The latest update of Radiation Therapy Oncology Group 91–11 with a median follow-up of 10.8 years continues to demonstrate higher larynx-preservation rates with combined CRT over the other modalities.[7]

Nowadays, CRT is a commonly used approach for the primary treatment of locally advanced laryngeal and nonlaryngeal HNC. This treatment strategy has demonstrated good locoregional control and survival outcomes when compared with historical surgical series.[9–11] However, these outcomes have been associated with a higher incidence of acute toxicity, such as mucositis and xerostomia.[12] In recent years, there has been more concern and awareness of the potential long-term toxicity, functional sequelae, and quality of life with the use of these treatment modalities.

Functional outcomes depend on multiple factors, including site of origin, stage of the cancer, treatment modality, baseline function, comorbidities, and quality of rehabilitation. Organ-preservation treatment does not always equal function preservation in HNC and can induce functional changes in quality of voice, speech, and swallowing and contribute to the quality of life of the patient.[13,14]

DEFINITION: WHAT IS THE FUNCTION OF THE LARYNX?

The primary and most primitive function of the larynx is to protect the lower airway. It is also responsible for voice production and plays a fundamental role in the speech and swallowing process. Therefore, it impacts communication, social interaction, personality, oral nutrition and hydration, and risk of aspiration.

Voice is defined as the sound originating from the vibration of the vocal cords/folds. The quality of the voice depends on the myoelastic characteristics of the vocal folds, and is also affected by the resonances and characteristics of the vocal tract. Speech is based on the volitional coordinated movements of the articulators and can be affected severely by changes in muscle or tissue properties (tongue or soft palate). In nonlaryngeal tumors, the tumor itself usually does not affect vocal fold vibration (ie, phonation), although depending on its location, it can impact vocal quality and speech production. In patients with laryngeal tumors, the tumor can have a negative effect on voicing, whereas its treatment can affect voice and speech. However, reported outcomes often combine both of these end points across multiple tumor sites and are not consistent in separating speech and voice outcomes.[15]

Dysphagia is difficulty swallowing safely or efficiently. It can lead to weight loss, malnutrition, and aspiration and its related complications. Swallowing includes four discrete phases: (1) the oral preparatory, (2) oral, (3) pharyngeal, and (4) esophageal stages. These four biomechanical events occur in a predictable sequence, and each stage is based on the movement patterns and timely occurrence of neurologic triggers from the previous stage.[16]

Normal speech and swallowing require precise coordination of a series of rapid, complex neuromuscular actions. Speech production is affected primarily by tumors that involve the tongue or subsites of the oral cavity. Swallowing can be affected by any cancer within the aerodigestive tract.[17] Any alteration in oral cavity, oropharyngeal or laryngeal structures, or their neural innervation that disrupt these neuromuscular patterns has some effect on speech and swallowing.

This article evaluates and summarizes the evidence-based medicine outcomes of recently published studies of laryngeal function after RT or CRT.

PHYSIOPATHOLOGY

It is uniformly recognized that the functional outcomes following optimal RT or CRT are usually good to excellent.[18–20] Indeed, it is often the treatment of choice for laryngeal cancers because the functional outcomes are good and seem superior to surgical management.[21,22] Although oncologically effective, radiation to the vocal folds can be associated with functional limitations. A fibroblastic response related to acute oxidative injury with resulting cell damage, ischemia, and inflammatory response has been hypothesized.[23] Despite these changes in some patients, the loss of vocal fold pliability chronically related to radiation fibrosis is thought to lead to hoarseness, inability to be heard over noise, and vocal strain with communication. The morbidity from radiation to the vocal folds for glottic larynx tumors has been described extensively and more recent data have also confirmed some decreased laryngeal function following radiation for nonglottic head and neck tumors.[24]

Berg and colleagues[25] reported the pathologic effects of external-beam irradiation on human vocal folds. A blinded, controlled study of archived tissue, postirradiation salvage laryngectomy vocal fold tissue was evaluated. Irradiated tissue was compared with nonirradiated benign control tissue. Histomorphometric analysis was used to assess muscle and collagen organization, superficial lamina propia (SLP) and vocal ligament thickness, vocalis muscle fiber area, collagen content, and hyaluronic acid. Immunohistochemical analyses were used to assess the content of type I collagen, type IV collagen, vimentin, fibronectin, α-smooth muscle actin, matrix metalloproteinase 9, and laminin. Twenty irradiated vocal folds were evaluated and compared with control specimens. Collagen and muscle disorganization was noted in the irradiated specimens. The SLP and vocal ligament thicknesses and the mean muscle fiber diameters did not differ significantly. The SLP fibronectin and the vocalis muscle and SLP collagen content were significantly increased in the irradiated vocal folds and the SLP collagen content increased significantly with time between irradiation and resection. The laminin content of irradiated vocalis muscles was significantly decreased. These vocal fold tissue changes can affect the vibration of the vocal folds and impact voice quality following RT.

Johns and colleagues[23] reported a translational study of radiation fibrosis of the vocal fold using archived human and fresh murine irradiated vocal fold tissue. Whole genome microarray analysis demonstrated increased transcription of markers for fibrosis, oxidative stress, inflammation, glycosaminoglycan production, and apoptosis. Irradiated vocal folds had increases in collagen and fibronectin transcription and deposition in the lamina propia. They reported that human and murine vocal fold tissue have similar changes leading to fibrosis that underlie loss of vocal fold pliability occurring in patients following laryngeal irradiation suggesting the potential benefit of using the mouse model in creating new prevention and treatment strategies for vocal fold radiation fibrosis.

Fibrosis has been considered the cause of late CRT-induced dysphagia for many years. Dysregulation of normal wound healing mechanisms, coupled with regional oxidative stress, may lead to overproduction of transforming growth factor-β1, which is a commonly studied and implicated regulator of the fibrotic process.[26] The fibrosis process is self-inducing and may spread to adjacent regions, accounting for the chronic and often progressive clinical presentation of fibrosis after RT. In addition, neuropathy can occur as the result of neural tumor infiltration, chemotoxicity, or as a late effect of RT, but in clinical practice it has been considered a less common cause of dysphagia.[27]

Preliminary data from the National Institutes of Health Laryngeal Study Section have expanded the understanding of neuromuscular cause of chronic dysphagia after CRT.[28] The authors found electromyographic evidence of at least partial denervation of the suprahyoid musculature (geniohyoid and mylohyoid) and the thyroid muscle, required to achieve supraglottic closure and upper esophageal opening, in 90% of nonsurgical patients enrolled in a trial for chronic dysphagia after RT or CRT for HNC. Also, intramuscular stimulation at rest induced hyolaryngeal movement similar to that of healthy control subjects, implying that the muscles in these dysphagia patients with HNC were not completely stiffened and fibrotic. Rather, a combination of denervation and muscle fibrosis was suggested. The cause of neuropathy after CRT is not fully understood, but brainstem neurotoxicity, nerve-induced damage, peripheral devascularization, and compressive injury from adjacent fibrosis may all be implicated.[28]

DIAGNOSIS OF LARYNGEAL DYSFUNCTION AFTER RADIATION THERAPY

To analyze the effects of the tumor versus the effects of radiation, pretreatment data are needed for a proper analysis of the various factors involved. In a systematic review reported by Jacobi and colleagues[15] only two studies were found to have a distinction between the effects of tumor versus treatment on voice and/or speech outcome. Kazi and colleagues[22] reported that laryngeal tumors distort voice quality because they obstruct the airflow through the glottis, they impair normal fold movement, and they are accompanied by significant edema. The treatment effects could be radiation-induced fibrosis or vocal fold atrophy and swelling of laryngeal and pharyngeal tissues. Meleca and colleagues[29] mentioned that vocal fold neuromuscular weakness and paresis could be a result of the invasive effects of the tumor, whereas fibrosis, mucositis of the laryngeal soft tissues, and vocal fold atrophic changes are caused by the treatment.

Impaired baseline functioning has been associated with suboptimal functional outcomes after organ-preservation therapy modalities, particularly higher levels of feeding tube dependence and tracheostomy in those patients with baseline aspiration of thin liquids[30] or vocal fold fixation[31,32] before RT. In two retrospective studies, the rates of chronic feeding tube or tracheostomy dependence were 35% to 56% in patients with baseline vocal fold fixation versus 6% in patients without fixation. Furthermore, recovery of vocal fold mobility after CRT was reported in 65% (52% full and 13% partial recovery) of patients with baseline fixation.[32] The recovery of vocal fold mobility after CRT was associated with significantly higher 5-year overall survival and local control and lower rates of persistent feeding tube and tracheostomy dependence.

The prognostic significance of baseline functioning supports the routine use of instrumental examination using laryngeal videostroboscopy and a modified barium swallowing study or flexible endoscopic evaluation of swallowing before CRT.

Evaluating and measuring swallowing and voice dysfunction after CRT greatly impacts outcomes reported in clinical studies. Different methods had been implicated, such as endoscopic swallowing studies, videofluoroscopic swallowing studies, and laryngeal videostroboscopy, to directly observe physiologic functioning during swallowing or voice production. The validated measures obtained by instrumental examinations are commonly considered the gold standard because they are more objective than a clinical evaluation of swallowing or patient self-report. There are also several psychometrically validated patient-reported outcome measures (eg, MD Anderson Dysphagia Inventory,[33] MD Anderson Symptom Inventory,[34] University of Washington Quality of Life Scale,[35] and Functional Assessment of Cancer Therapy-Head and Neck) that are available to assess functioning and provide a complementary evaluation and perspective at a lower cost option. Other indicators of functional status, such as diet level, gastrostomy, and tracheostomy dependence, are commonly used in clinic to evaluate the function because they are simple measures to collect and interpret.

VOICE OUTCOMES

In early stage larynx cancer, Harrison and colleagues[36] reported a prospective computer-assisted voice analysis: the functional result of laryngeal irradiation. Twenty-five patients underwent vocal analysis using a voice analyzer interfaced with a computer allowing for the determination of percent voicing (%V; normal = presence of phonation = 90–100%V). Other parameters, such as breathiness (air turbulence or hoarseness) and strain (vocal cord tension), were also measured. Patients were recorded before RT, weekly during RT, and at set intervals after RT. All patients had local control and demonstrated normal phonation pattern by 3 months after RT, and was sustained at 9 months follow-up. In addition, 94% of patients have had significant decrease in breathiness after RT, which objectively documents diminished hoarseness. In 83%, breathiness was normal after RT. Most patients have had increased strain after RT, which documents increased vocal cord tension, but strain remained within normal limits in 89%. This analysis suggested that most patients irradiated for early glottic cancer demonstrate a decrease in breathiness and an increase in strain after RT, and enjoy a resultant voice that has normal phonation maintained at 9 months after RT.

Our group also reported the functional outcomes and patterns of failure for T1-T2 glottic cancer after definitive RT.[37] A total of 253 patients with early glottic cancer underwent two- or three-dimensional RT to a median dose of 63 Gy in 2.25 Gy per fraction. After a median follow-up of 83 months, the locoregional control for the whole cohort was 98% and the 5-year cause-specific survival was 100% with remarkable functional preservation and negligible long-term toxicity. We also investigated the impact of definitive RT in early glottic cancer on clinical outcomes, particularly in

RT-induced dysphagia and carotid vasculopathy,[38] showing that the mean dose to critical structures (larynx, pharyngeal constrictors, and carotid arteries) and their volume size can be predictors of better functional outcomes and advocating that such techniques as intensity-modulated RT (IMRT) can provide a finest planning target volume coverage with lower doses to the organs at risk and potentially continuing to improve these functional outcomes.[39]

Al-Mamgani and colleagues[40] published the outcomes for T1-T2 glottic cancer treated with RT in a series of 1050 patients and a prospective assessment of quality of life and voice handicap index in a subset of 233 patients. In this study, they found excellent outcomes with good quality of life and voice handicap index scores except in the subset of patients with T2b tumors or those who continued smoking after RT, advocating the importance of the bulkiness of the disease and smoking cessation in the ultimate voice functional outcome after RT.

It is known that locally advanced laryngeal cancer is frequently treated with CRT but can increase the risk of laryngeal edema and dysfunction. In contrast, RT without chemotherapy, delivered to small fields for early stage glottic larynx cancer, usually results in excellent voice quality.[41] Sanguineti and colleagues[42] found that neck stage, nodal diameter, mean laryngeal dose, and percentage of laryngeal volume receiving greater than or equal to 50 Gy were all significantly associated with laryngeal edema grade 2 or greater suggesting that the mean laryngeal dose should be kept as low as possible, ideally less than 44 Gy, to obtain better functional outcomes.

Speech and voice outcomes can also be affected based on glottic versus supraglottic larynx RT. Dornfeld and colleagues[43] found a strong correlation between speech and doses delivered to the aryepiglottic folds, pre-epiglottic space, false vocal cords, and lateral pharyngeal walls at the level of the false vocal cords. In particular, they noted a steep decrease in function after 66 Gy to these structures. Other evidence suggests that saliva, pharyngeal lubrication, soft tissue and structural changes within the surrounding musculature, initial tumor size and volume, and tumor shrinkage and response play an important role in the voice outcome.[24,44]

Recently, Aaltonen and colleagues[45] reported the outcomes in voice quality of a randomized trial comparing laser surgery with RT for the treatment of early vocal cord cancer. Voice quality was assessed at baseline and 6 and 24 months after treatment. The main outcome measures were expert-rated voice quality on the GRBAS (Grade, Roughness, Breathiness, Asthenia, Strain) scale, videolaryngostroboscopic findings, and the patients' self-rated voice quality and its impact on activities of daily living. Overall voice quality between the groups was rated similar, but voice was more breathy and the glottal gap was wider in patients treated with laser surgery. Patients treated with RT reported less hoarseness-related inconvenience in daily living 2 years after treatment, suggesting that RT may be the treatment of choice for patients whose requirements for voice quality are demanding or who want to maximize their functional outcome.

In nonlaryngeal tumors, Fung and colleagues[24] reported a comparison study of vocal function following radiation for nonlaryngeal versus laryngeal tumors of the head and neck. This retrospective study evaluated subjective and objective parameters of vocal function in patients irradiated to the head and neck with acoustic analyses, aerodynamic measurements, and videostroboscopy. All subjects were men, smokers, and treated 12 months or prior. They used the Voice Handicap Index (VHI) for self-assessment of voice quality. A total of 30 patients were evaluated, 17 with nonlaryngeal tumors and 13 with early glottic tumors. Acoustic parameters were worse for 75% of the acoustic measures of vowel production in the nonlaryngeal group. These include jitter, relative amplitude perturbation (shimmer), amplitude perturbation quotient, normalized noise energy, pitch amplitude, and spectral flatness ratio. Acoustic analyses revealed no difference in fundamental frequency. All aerodynamic measures, including mean phonation time and mean airflow, were decreased in the nonlaryngeal group. Videostroboscopy demonstrated increased supraglottic activity in the nonlaryngeal group. Voice handicap was significantly greater in the nonlaryngeal group. The conclusion of the study was that when compared with patients receiving RT for early glottic tumors, there is objective and subjective evidence of vocal dysfunction in patients treated with wide-field RT for nonlaryngeal tumors.

The consensus recommendations for functional assessment in laryngeal-preservation trials suggest the use of simple, validated scales to assess vocal outcomes.[46] The ones commonly used are the Voice-Related Quality of Life and the VHI, or its abbreviated version, the VHI-10.[47,48]

In 2009, a cross-sectional study[49] compared voice outcomes of 137 patients with laryngeal cancer using these two scales along with the clinician-rated auditory-perceptual scale GRBAS scale. Most patients were early glottic cancers, and outcomes were stratified for comparison into four groups by final treatment modality: (1) RT alone, (2) RT with concurrent platinum chemotherapy, (3) laser surgery, or (4) total laryngectomy. At a median of 38 months, a similar trend was seen across the three voice outcome measures (VHI-10, Voice-Related Quality of Life, and GRBAS). Patients treated with RT and CRT had similar results on each outcome measure. Superior voice outcomes were identified in patients treated with RT alone and CRT, followed by laser surgery. Voice outcomes were uniformly lowest in patients treated with total laryngectomy. The authors considered the effect of time after treatment and found that few patients treated with RT or CRT experienced significantly diminished vocal functioning as a late effect of treatment.

DYSPHAGIA OUTCOMES

The prevalence of dysphagia after CRT depends on the duration of follow-up and outcome measure reported. In 2010, Francis and colleagues[50] reported population-based estimates of swallowing outcomes from SEER-Medicare data in 8002 patients with oral, pharyngeal, and laryngeal squamous cell carcinomas. The primary swallow outcomes evaluated were dysphagia, stricture, and pneumonia with rates of 64%, 12%, and 15%, respectively. The highest were for those treated with CRT compared with other modalities including surgery with adjuvant RT. Patients on CRT were 44% more likely to develop pneumonia after treatment than patients who underwent surgery alone. The results of the study provide evidence that suggests that swallowing outcomes in HNC survivors are more adversely affected by CRT than by other treatment modalities despite that the authors of the study acknowledged the unknown sensitivity of diagnostic and procedural codes to capture asymptomatic dysphagia (silent aspiration) limiting the data analysis.

Feeding Tube Dependence

The most common swallowing outcome reported is the rate of feeding tube dependence. However, this may underestimate the rates of dysphagia because patients often eat despite evidence of dysphagia or aspiration. There are multiple clinical trials of RT or CRT for HNC that reported low rates of patients feeding tube dependant, particularly those treated with IMRT in a comprehensive HNC center.

Mourad and colleagues[51] reported the oncologic and functional outcomes of a series of patients with locally advanced tonsillar cancer treated at the Institute for Head, Neck and Thyroid Cancer in New York. Of 79 patients, most were stage III-IV disease, with

95% locoregional control at 5 years and only 4% percutaneous endoscopic gastrostomy tube dependency.

Other series, including the ones from University of Florida,[52] Princess Margaret Hospital,[53] and University of Michigan,[54] had reported functional outcomes after treatment of oropharyngeal cancers with RT or CRT, with rates less than 5% of feeding tube dependency and with excellent locoregional control and survival outcomes.

Aspiration

Patients on treatment with CRT for HNC are commonly evaluated for aspiration. The reported rates differ because of the sensitivity of the different examination instruments to report silent aspiration in asymptomatic patients who do not report dysphagia. An important consideration for the interpretation of the reported data is that many clinicians only perform swallowing studies in symptomatic patients who complain of dysphagia after CRT resulting in a bias and underestimation of the results. It is important to be aware and recognize that aspiration has been documented in 68% to 81% of patients before or after CRT of the head and neck, as detected with modified swallowing barium study.[55]

Silent aspiration has been observed in at least one-third of aspirators after CRT.[56,57] When aspiration rates were only reported in symptomatic patients evaluated using instrumental swallowing studies after CRT the reported rate varies from 24% to 31%.[58] In contrast, studies that reported rates of symptomatic and asymptomatic aspiration with instrumental swallowing evaluations report higher aspiration rates of 30% to 62%.[59,60]

Stricture

An important contributor to dysphagia after CRT for HNC is pharyngoesophageal stricture. Stricture is not as common as physiologic impairments that reduce the range of motion of swallowing structures; however, when it develops it can greatly impact the swallowing function and lead to prolonged feeding tube dependence.[30]

Reported stricture rates after CRT for laryngeal and pharyngeal cancer range from 12% to 37%.[61–63] Higher rates of stricture had been reported particularly in patients treated for hypopharynx cancer and after CRT regimens with a hyperfractionated regimen.[50,61] Patient-specific factors that predispose to stricture formation had been identified. Duration of mucositis has been implicated as an independent risk factor for stricture with a 32% increased risk with each week of mucositis.[63]

In a prospective study, there was significant correlation between the occurrence of aspiration and the mean dose to the pharyngeal constrictors and larynx. The volume of larynx and inferior constrictors receiving greater than or equal to 50 Gy were statistically associated with aspiration and stricture, and the mean larynx dose was statistically associated with aspiration.[62,64] Dose to the superior constrictor has also been found to be strongly significant.[65] Dose-volume analysis presented dose-volume parameters for the inferior pharyngeal constrictor and cricoid pharyngeal inlet that would decrease the risk of dysphagia and feeding tube as follows: inferior pharyngeal constrictor V65, less than 15%; inferior pharyngeal constrictor V60, less than 40%; inferior pharyngeal constrictor mean, less than 55 Gy; and cricoid pharyngeal inlet maximum dose, less than 60 Gy.[56] In another study, the probability of a swallowing disorder increased 19% per 10 Gy after 55 Gy to the superior constrictor muscle. With a mean dose of 51, 48, and 32 Gy to the superior, middle, and inferior constrictor muscles, respectively, an overall probability of incidences of 2%, 10%, 20%, and 50% were estimated at 22, 44, 55, and 74 Gy to the superior constrictor muscle using a logistic model.

Quality of Life

Nguyen and colleagues[66] reported that the degree of anxiety, depression, and compromised quality of life that patients with HNC can experience after treatment is correlated with the severity of their dysphagia. In that study, it was shown that patients with aspiration who required prolonged tube feedings had the worst quality of life.

STRATEGIES FOR PREVENTION OF LARYNGEAL DYSFUNCTION

Many studies have shown the efficacy of preventive and rehabilitative strategies to improve laryngeal function outcomes. Referral to a speech and swallowing pathologist before treatment is a key component of the multidisciplinary management of these patients.

Risk reduction may be achieved by de-escalating treatment intensity in cancers with favorable survival rates (eg, human papillomavirus positive). Different methods have been considered to reduce treatment intensity, including risk-based treatment planning, targeted therapy, and IMRT. Multiple data have demonstrated an association between dose and volume coverage to organs at risk with IMRT (eg, oral cavity, constrictor muscles, and larynx) and swallowing and speech and voice outcomes.[67,68]

Our group reported the outcomes of a prospective cohort using a de-escalating treatment modality with unilateral RT for node-positive human papillomavirus–positive squamous cell carcinoma of the tonsil.[69] Twenty-three patients, most with T2 N2b disease, were treated with unilateral neck irradiation. With a median follow-up of 24 months, there were no contralateral neck failures, 100% locoregional control, only two patients with xerostomia grade 2, and no patient dependent on percutaneous endoscopic gastrostomy tube.

Regardless of the method used to deintensify therapy, instrumental swallowing examinations are needed to comprehensively evaluate swallowing outcomes. Early intervention benefits functional outcomes. Preventive swallowing therapy encourages use of swallowing musculature during treatment by avoiding periods of no oral intake and adherence to targeted swallowing exercises.[70,71] The swallow exercise regimens have been associated with superior swallowing-related quality-of-life scores,[72] improved swallowing function (better base of tongue retraction and epiglottic inversion),[73] larger post-RT muscle mass (genioglossus, mylohyoid, and hyoglossus), T2 signal intensity on MRI,[74] and shorter duration of feeding tube dependence after RT.[75]

Knowing the relationship between xerostomia and dysphagia,[76] RT techniques that improve salivary gland function, such as parotid gland–sparing conformal RT or IMRT,[77,78] can reduce rates of xerostomia and dysphagia. A mean radiation dose to the parotid gland of 26 Gy or less should be the goal.[79]

Eisbruch and colleagues[64] reported dysphagia and aspiration after CRT for HNC: which anatomic structures are affected and can they be spare by IMRT? Dysphagia-aspiration–related structures including the superior, middle, and inferior pharyngeal constrictor muscles; the cricopharyngeal muscle; the esophagus; and the glottis and supraglottis can be damaged and can cause dysphagia and aspiration. IMRT can reduce the doses to the dysphagia-aspiration–related structures and data have been shown that there needs to be a reduction in the mean doses and volumes of the dysphagia-aspiration–related structures that receive 50 Gy or more.[65,80–82]

Other strategies, such as swallowing exercises (eg, range of motion exercises, resistance exercises), are recommended pretreatment to improve functional outcomes.[17] Swallowing maneuvers including Mendelsohn maneuver, supraglottic swallow, super-supraglottic swallow, and effortful swallow can be used to improve swallowing.[83,84]

In some cases, surgical treatment (eg, dilation) may be needed. However, the cause of the dysphagia must be confirmed via clinical examination and diagnostic studies to rule out the possibility of cancer recurrence as the cause of any progressive dysphagia.

SUMMARY

Organ and function preservation are not necessarily synonymous. In general, the preference of CRT over surgery combined with RT seems to be justified in locally advanced HNCs, although there are still potential negative effects. Technical improvements in RT planning and delivery have improved outcomes considerably. Further improvements are expected as the treatments are deintensified.

Functional preservation is a key aspect and focus of contemporary HNC management. Current evidence clearly documents high rates of locoregional control and reasonably good swallowing and voice outcome after CRT for laryngeal and pharyngeal cancers. The data suggest more favorable voice outcomes for primary RT compared with conservation surgery or total laryngectomy for glottic cancers. Awareness of the radiation targeted areas and dose tolerances of organs at risk (oral cavity, constrictor muscles, larynx) in combination with newer radiation techniques, such as IMRT/IGRT (image-guided radiation therapy) or proton therapy, are strategies to minimize the prevalence of swallowing dysfunction after RT, with promising results. Consensus and newer validated methods are needed to have a better and more standardize form to evaluate functional outcomes, particularly for those patients with an impaired baseline function. The analysis of functional outcomes should be included in phase III organ-preservation trials to allow reliable comparisons among treatment regimens.

Newer deintensification treatment strategies and more personalized treatments are helpful to continue improved functional outcomes in patients with HNC. It is clear that the evaluation and management of these patients should be with an experienced multidisciplinary team to obtain the best outcomes. Preventive voice, speech, and swallowing therapy had shown a critical role to reduce the rates of dysfunction after CRT.

Investigation regarding laryngeal fibrosis caused by other etiologies provides several possible interventions including mesenchymal stem cells and growth factor therapy, or the use of pharmacologic therapy with pentoxifylline and vitamin E. With an improved understanding of critical biochemical changes following radiation, potential targets for intervention can be developed to prevent and/or treat radiation-induced fibrosis.

A baseline evaluation of speech and swallowing function is critical and recommended for the prediction of posttreatment functioning. There is a significant need for research in this field to implement new strategies and improve existing strategies to obtain continued improvements in the functional outcomes of these patients.

REFERENCES

1. Jemal A, Bray F, Center MM, et al. Global cancer statistics. CA Cancer J Clin 2011;61:69–90.
2. Siegel R, Ma J, Zou Z, et al. Cancer statistics 2014. CA Cancer J Clin 2014;64: 9–29.
3. Harrison LB, Sessions RB, Merrill SK. Head and neck cancer: a multidisciplinary approach. 4th edition. Philadelphia: Wolters Kluwer/Lippincott Williams and Wilkins; 2013. p. 441–59.

4. DeSanto LW, Olsen KD, Perry WC, et al. Quality of life after surgical treatment of cancer of the larynx. Ann Otol Rhinol Laryngol 1995;104:763–9.
5. Induction chemotherapy plus radiation compared with surgery plus radiation in patients with advanced laryngeal cancer. The Department of Veterans Affairs Laryngeal Cancer Study Group. N Engl J Med 1991;324:1685–90.
6. Forastiere AA, Goepfert H, Maor M, et al. Concurrent chemotherapy and radiotherapy for organ preservation in advanced laryngeal cancer. N Engl J Med 2003;349:2091–8.
7. Forastiere AA, Zhang Q, Weber RS, et al. Long-term results of RTOG 91-11: a comparison of three nonsurgical treatment strategies to preserve the larynx in patients with locally advanced larynx cancer. J Clin Oncol 2013;31:845–52.
8. Pfister DG, Strong E, Harrison LB, et al. Larynx preservation with combined chemotherapy and radiation therapy in advanced but resectable head and neck cancer. J Clin Oncol 1991;9:850–9.
9. Pfister DG, Laurie SA, Weinstein GS, et al. American Society of Clinical Oncology clinical practice guideline for the use of larynx-preservation strategies in the treatment of laryngeal cancer. J Clin Oncol 2006;24:3693–704.
10. Chen AY, Scharag N, Hao Y, et al. Changes in the treatment of advanced laryngeal cancer 1985–2001. Otolaryngol Head Neck Surg 2006;135:831–7.
11. Pignon JP, le Maitre A, Maillard E, et al. Meta-analysis of chemotherapy in head and neck cancer (MACH-NC): an update on 93 randomised trials and 17,346 patients. Radiother Oncol 2009;92:4–14.
12. Trotti A, Bellm LA, Epstein JB, et al. Mucositis incidence, severity and associated outcomes in patients with head and neck cancer receiving radiotherapy with or without chemotherapy: a systematic literature review. Radiother Oncol 2003;66:253–62.
13. Peeters AJ, van Gogh CD, Goor KM, et al. Health status and voice outcome after treatment for T1a glottic carcinoma. Eur Arch Otorhinolaryngol 2004;261:534–40.
14. Fung K, Yoo J, Leeper HA, et al. Effects of head and neck radiation therapy on vocal function. J Otolaryngol 2001;30:133–9.
15. Jacobi I, Van der Molen L, Huiskens H, et al. Voice and speech outcomes of chemoradiation for advanced head and neck cancer: a systematic review. Eur Arch Otorhinolaryngol 2010;267:1495–505.
16. Bhandare N, Mendenhall WM. A literature review of late complications of radiation therapy for head and neck cancers: incidence and dose response. J Nucl Med Radiat Ther 2012. Available online at: http://dx.doi.org/10.4172/2155-9619.S2-009.
17. Mittal BB, Pauloski BR, Haraf DJ, et al. Swallowing dysfunction-preventive and rehabilitation strategies in patients with head-and-neck cancers treated with surgery, radiotherapy, and chemotherapy: a critical review. Int J Radiat Oncol Biol Phys 2003;57:1219–30.
18. Pfister DG, Harrison LB, Strong EW, et al. Organ-function preservation in advanced oropharynx cancer: results with induction chemotherapy and radiation. J Clin Oncol 1995;13:671–80.
19. Myers C, Kerr P, Cooke A, et al. Functional outcomes after treatment of advanced oropharyngeal carcinoma with radiation or chemoradiation. J Otolaryngol Head Neck Surg 2012;41:108–18.
20. Hutcheson KA, Lewin JS, Holsinger FC, et al. Long-term functional and survival outcomes after induction chemotherapy and risk-based definitive therapy for locally advanced squamous cell carcinoma of the head and neck. Head Neck 2014;36:474–80.

21. Fung K, Lyden TH, Lee J, et al. Voice and swallowing outcomes of an organ-preservation trial for advanced laryngeal cancer. Int J Radiat Oncol Biol Phys 2005;63:1395–9.
22. Kazi R, Venkitaraman R, Johnson C, et al. Electroglottographic comparison of voice outcomes in patients with advanced laryngopharyngeal cancer treated by chemoradiotherapy or total laryngectomy. Int J Radiat Oncol Biol Phys 2008;70:344–52.
23. Johns MM, Kolachala V, Berg E, et al. Radiation fibrosis of the vocal fold: from man to mouse. Laryngoscope 2012;122:S107–25.
24. Fung K, Yoo J, Leeper HA, et al. Vocal function following radiation for non-laryngeal versus laryngeal tumors of the head and neck. Laryngoscope 2001;111:1920–4.
25. Berg EE, Kolachala V, Branski RC, et al. Pathologic effects of external-beam irradiation on human vocal folds. Ann Otol Rhinol Laryngol 2011;120:748–54.
26. Martin M, Lefaix J, Delanian S. TGF-beta1 and radiation fibrosis: a master switch and a specific therapeutic target? Int J Radiat Oncol Biol Phys 2000;47:277–90.
27. Hutcheson KA, Lewin JS. Functional outcomes after chemoradiotherapy of laryngeal and pharyngeal cancers. Curr Oncol Rep 2012;14:158–65.
28. Martin S, Chung B, Bratlund C, et al. Movement trajectories during percutaneous simulation at rest of the hyolaryngeal muscles in head and neck cancer patients treated with radiation therapy. Dysphagia 2010;25:354–98.
29. Meleca RJ, Dworkin JP, Kewson DT, et al. Functional outcomes following nonsurgical treatment for advanced-stage laryngeal carcinoma. Laryngoscope 2003;113:720–8.
30. Hutcheson KA, Barringer DA, Rosenthal DI, et al. Swallowing outcomes after radiotherapy for laryngeal carcinoma. Arch Otolaryngol Head Neck Surg 2008;134:178–83.
31. Staton J, Robbins KT, Newman L, et al. Factors predictive of poor functional outcome after chemoradiation for advanced laryngeal cancer. Otolaryngol Head Neck Surg 2002;127:43–7.
32. Solares CA, Wood B, Rodriguez CP, et al. Does vocal cord fixation preclude nonsurgical management of laryngeal cancer? Laryngoscope 2009;119:1130–4.
33. Chen AY, Frankowski R, Bishop-Leone J, et al. The development and validation of a dysphagia-specific quality-of-life questionnaire for patients with head and neck cancer: the M.D. Anderson dysphagia inventory. Arch Otolaryngol Head Neck Surg 2001;127:870–6.
34. Rosenthal DI, Mendoza TR, Chambers MS, et al. Measuring head and neck cancer symptom burden: the development and validation of the M.D. Anderson symptom inventory, head and neck module. Head Neck 2007;29:923–31.
35. Rogers SN, Gwanne S, Lowe D, et al. The addition of mood and anxiety domains to the University of Washington quality of life scale. Head Neck 2002;24:521–9.
36. Harrison LB, Solomon B, Miller S, et al. Prospective computer-assisted voice analysis for patients with early stage glottic cancer: a preliminary report of the functional result of laryngeal irradiation. Int J Radiat Oncol Biol Phys 1990;19:123–7.
37. Mourad WF, Hu KS, Shourbaji RA, et al. Long-term follow-up and pattern of failure for T1-T2 glottic cancer after definitive radiation therapy. Am J Clin Oncol 2013;36:580–3.
38. Mourad WF, Shasha D, Blakaj DM, et al. Comprehensive head and neck radiotherapy dose-volume constraints do not apply to smaller volumes. Anticancer Res 2013;33:4483–9.

39. Mourad WF, Hu KS, Shourbaji RA, et al. Exploration of the role of radiotherapy in the management of early glottic cancer with complete carotid artery occlusion. Onkologie 2013;36:433–5.
40. Al-Mamgani A, Van Rooij PH, Woutersen DP, et al. Radiotherapy for T1-2N0 glottic cancer: a multivariate analysis of predictive factors for the long-term outcome in 1050 patients and a prospective assessment of quality of life and voice handicap index in a subset of 233 patients. Clin Otolaryngol 2013;38:306–12.
41. Fu KK, Woofhouse RJ, Quivey JM, et al. The significance of laryngeal edema following radiotherapy of carcinoma of the vocal cord. Cancer 1982;49:6555–8.
42. Sanguineti G, Adapala P, Endres EJ, et al. Dosimetric predictors of laryngeal edema. Int J Radiat Oncol Biol Phys 2007;68:741–9.
43. Dornfeld K, Simmons JR, Karnell L, et al. Radiation doses to structures within and adjacent to the larynx are correlated with long-term diet and speech-related quality of life. Int J Radiat Oncol Biol Phys 2007;68:750–7.
44. Rancati T, Schwarz M, Allen AM, et al. Radiation dose-volume effects in the larynx and pharynx. Int J Radiat Oncol Biol Phys 2010;76:S64–9.
45. Aaltonen LM, Rautiainen N, Sellman J, et al. Voice quality after treatment of early vocal cord cancer: a randomized trial comparing laser surgery with radiation therapy. Int J Radiat Oncol Biol Phys 2014;90:255–60.
46. Ang KK. Larynx preservation clinical trial design: summary of key recommendations of a consensus panel. Oncologist 2010;15(Suppl 3):25–9.
47. Hogikyan ND, Sethuraman G. Validation of an instrument to measure voice-related quality of life (V-RQOL). J Voice 1999;13:557–69.
48. Rosen CA, Lee AS, Osborne J, et al. Development and validation of the voice handicap index-10. Laryngoscope 2004;114:1549–56.
49. Oridate N, Homma A, Suzuki S, et al. Voice-related quality of life after treatment of laryngeal cancer. Arch Otolaryngol Head Neck Surg 2009;135:363–8.
50. Francis DO, Weymuller EA Jr, Parvathaneni U, et al. Dysphagia, stricture, and pneumonia in head and neck cancer patients: does treatment modality matter? Ann Otol Rhinol Laryngol 2010;119:391–7.
51. Mourad WF, Hu K, Harrison LB, et al. Five-year outcomes of squamous cell carcinoma of the tonsil treated with radiotherapy. Am J Clin Oncol 2014;37:57–62.
52. Mendenhall WM, Morris CG, Amdur RJ, et al. Definitive radiotherapy for tonsillar squamous cell carcinoma. Am J Clin Oncol 2006;29:290–7.
53. O'Sullivan B, Warde P, Grice B, et al. The benefits and pitfalls of ipsilateral radiotherapy in carcinoma of the tonsillar region. Int J Radiat Oncol Biol Phys 2001;51:332–43.
54. Eisbruch A, Harris J, Garden AS, et al. Multi-institutional trial of accelerated hypofractionated intensity-modulated radiation therapy for early stage oropharyngeal cancer (RTOG 00-22). Int J Radiat Oncol Biol Phys 2010;76:1333–8.
55. Nguyen NP, Smith HJ, Sallah S, et al. Evaluation and management of swallowing dysfunction following chemoradiation for head and neck cancer. Curr Opin Otolaryngol Head Neck Surg 2007;15:130–3.
56. Goguen LA, Posner MR, Norris CM, et al. Dysphagia after sequential chemoradiation therapy for advanced head and neck cancer. Otolaryngol Head Neck Surg 2006;134:916–22.
57. Nguyen NP, Moltz CC, Frank C, et al. Dysphagia following chemoradiation for locally advanced head and neck cancer. Ann Oncol 2004;15:383–8.
58. Caudell JJ, Schaner PE, Meredith RF, et al. Factors associated with long-term dysphagia after definitive radiotherapy for locally advanced head-and-neck cancer. Int J Radiat Oncol Biol Phys 2009;73:410–5.

59. Eisbruch A, Lyden T, Bradford CR, et al. Objective assessment of swallowing dysfunction and aspiration after radiation concurrent with chemotherapy for head-and-neck cancer. Int J Radiat Oncol Biol Phys 2002;53:23–8.

60. Agarwal J, Palwe V, Dutta D, et al. Objective assessment of swallowing function after definitive concurrent (chemo) radiotherapy in patients with head and neck cancer. Dysphagia 2011;26:399–406.

61. Lee WT, Akst LM, Adelstein DJ, et al. Risk factors for hypopharyngeal/upper esophageal stricture formation after concurrent chemoradiation. Head Neck 2006;28:808–12.

62. Caglar HB, Tishler RB, Othus M, et al. Dose to larynx predicts for swallowing complications after intensity-modulated radiotherapy. Int J Radiat Oncol Biol Phys 2008;72:1110–8.

63. Best SR, Ha PK, Blanco RG, et al. Factors associated with pharyngoesophageal stricture in patients treated with concurrent chemotherapy and radiation therapy for oropharyngeal squamous cell carcinoma. Head Neck 2011;33:1727–34.

64. Eisbruch A, Schwartz M, Rasch C, et al. Dysphagia and aspiration after chemo-radiotherapy for head-and-neck cancer: which anatomic structures are affected and can they be spared by IMRT? Int J Radiat Oncol Biol Phys 2004;60:1425–39.

65. Feng FY, Kim HM, Lydent TH, et al. Intensity modulated radiotherapy of head and neck cancer aiming to reduce dysphagia: early dose-effect relationships for the swallowing structures. Int J Radiat Oncol Biol Phys 2007;68:1289–98.

66. Nguyen NP, Frank C, Moltz CC, et al. Impact of dysphagia on quality of life after treatment of head-and-neck cancer. Int J Radiat Oncol Biol Phys 2005;61:772–8.

67. Boscolo-Rizzo P, Gava A, Marchiori C, et al. Functional organ preservation in patients with locoregionally advanced head and neck squamous cell carcinoma treated by platinum-based multidrug induction chemotherapy and concurrent chemoradiotherapy. Ann Oncol 2011;22:1894–901.

68. Schwartz DL, Hutcheson K, Barringer D, et al. Candidate dosimetric predictors of long-term swallowing dysfunction after oropharyngeal intentisty-modulated radio-therapy. Int J Radiat Oncol Biol Phys 2010;78:1356–65.

69. Gamez M, Hu K, Harrison L, et al. Unilateral radiation therapy for node-positive HPV-positive squamous cell carcinoma of the tonsil: analysis of a prospective cohort [abstract: 2766]. Int J Radiat Oncol Biol Phys 2014;90:S513.

70. Rosenthal DI, Lewin JS, Eisbruch A. Prevention and treatment of dysphagia and aspiration after chemoradiation for head and neck cancer. J Clin Oncol 2006;24: 2636–43.

71. Gillespie MB, Brodsky MB, Day TA, et al. Swallowing-related quality of life after head and neck cancer treatment. Laryngoscope 2004;114:1362–7.

72. Kullbersh BD, Rosenthal EL, McGrew BM, et al. Pretreatment, preoperative swallowing exercises may improve dysphagia quality of life. Laryngoscope 2006;116: 883–6.

73. Carroll WR, Locher JL, Canon CL, et al. Pretreament swallowing exercises improve swallow function after chemoradiation. Laryngoscope 2008;118:39–43.

74. Carnaby-Mann GC, Amdur R, Schmalfuss I. Preventive exercise for dysphagia following head/neck cancer [abstract]. Dysphagia 2007;22:381.

75. Bhayani M, Hutcheson KA, Barringer DA, et al. Gastrostomy tube placement in patients with hypopharyngeal cancer treated with chemoradiotherapy: factors affecting placement and dependence [abstract]. Dysphagia 2011;26:471.

76. Logemann JA, Pauloski BR, Rademaker AW, et al. Xerostomia: 12-month changes in saliva production and its relationship to perception and performance

of swallow function, oral intake, and diet after chemoradiation. Head Neck 2003; 25:432–7.

77. Chao KS, Deasy JO, Markman J, et al. A prospective study of salivary function sparing in patients with head-and-neck cancers receiving intensity-modulated or three-dimensional radiation therapy: initial results. Int J Radiat Oncol Biol Phys 2001;49:907–16.

78. Eisbruch A, Kim HM, Terrell JE, et al. Xerostomia and its predictors following parotid-sparing irradiation of head-and-neck cancer. Int J Radiat Oncol Biol Phys 2001;50:695–704.

79. Eisbruch A, Ten Haken RK, Kim HM, et al. Dose, volume, and function relationships in parotid salivary glands following conformal and intensity-modulated irradiation of head and neck cancer. Int J Radiat Oncol Biol Phys 1999;45:577–87.

80. Jensen K, Lambersten K, Grau C, et al. Late swallowing dysfunction and dysphagia after radiotherapy for pharynx cancer: frequency, intensity and correlation with dose and volume parameters. Radiother Oncol 2007;85:74–82.

81. Levendag PC, Teugh DN, Voet P, et al. Dysphagia disorders in patients with cancer of the oropharynx are significantly affected by the radiation therapy dose to the superior and middle constrictor muscle: a dose-effect relationship. Radiother Oncol 2007;85:64–73.

82. Eisbruch A, Levendag PC, Feng FY, et al. Can IMRT or brachytherapy reduce dysphagia associated with chemoradiotherapy of head and neck cancer? The Michigan and Rotterdam experiences. Int J Radiat Oncol Biol Phys 2007;69(2 Suppl):S40–2.

83. Martin BJ, Logemann JA, Shaker R, et al. Normal laryngeal valving patterns during three-breath hold maneuvers a pilot investigation. Dysphagia 1993;8:11–20.

84. Lazarus C, Logemann JA, Gibbons P. Effects of maneuvers on swallow functioning in a dysphagic oral cancer patient. Head Neck 1993;15:419–24.

Management of Dysphonia After Radiation Therapy

Craig R. Villari, MD[a], Mark S. Courey, MD[b],*

KEYWORDS

- Laryngeal cancer • Radiation • Dysphonia • Speech therapy
- Vocal fold augmentation

KEY POINTS

- Radiation of the larynx can lead to fibrosis and decreased mucosal wave propagation. These can result in changes of both subjective perception of and objective measures of voice.
- Speech therapy is the main treatment modality used for voice rehabilitation after radiation for early laryngeal malignancies. Therapy regimens designed to reduce inflammation and maintain or improve flexibility of voice may benefit patients who have received radiation.
- Surgical techniques addressing postradiation changes of the larynx are limited and have not been applied to large populations of affected patients.
- Further research is needed to more completely examine the role of behavioral, surgical, and pharmacologic intervention.

INTRODUCTION

To discuss rehabilitation of the irradiated larynx, a sound understanding of the physiology and function of the normal larynx and that of the irradiated larynx is required. These topics are covered elsewhere in this publication (see the articles by Niv Mor and Mauricio Gamez elsewhere in this issue). They serve as foundational building blocks for discussing behavioral, medical, and surgical intervention geared toward restoring the voice in the postradiation patient.

Radiation-induced dysphonia can develop after radiation therapy (RT) for a primary laryngeal cancer or when the larynx is in the radiation field for nonlaryngeal malignancy and cannot be, or is not, spared. Dysphonia related to radiation exposure appears to

The authors have no financial disclosures related to this content.
[a] Department of Otolaryngology-Head and Neck Surgery, Emory University Hospital, Midtown Medical Office Tower, Suite 1135, Atlanta, GA 30308, USA; [b] Department of Otolaryngology-Head and Neck Surgery, University of California – San Francisco, 2330 Post Street, 5th Floor, San Francisco, CA 94115, USA
* Corresponding author.
E-mail address: Mark.Courey@ucsf.edu

be dose dependent. In patients with nonlaryngeal primary head and neck malignancies, dysphonia becomes problematic when the dose to the larynx exceeds 50 Gy.[1] This dose is less than the treatment dose for laryngeal primary malignancies, but the resultant rate of dysphonia at this level of radiation exposure is unknown. Radiation is often chosen as a treatment modality for early laryngeal primary squamous cell carcinoma (T1 or T2 disease) given its excellent cure rates but usually requires doses in excess of 65 Gy.[2–5] Resultantly, between 14% and 92% of patients report dysphonia after radiotherapy for early laryngeal malignancies.[6–10]

The timing of the development of dysphonia after RT is variable. Patients can present with dysphonia early during treatment or they may have initial improvement in their voice only to worsen 5 to 15 or more years after treatment; those with early onset can persist for years or may improve spontaneously. Acute voice changes stem from oxidative injury resulting in injury to both diseased and normal tissue; this can lead to mucosal edema and necrosis and resultant epithelial sloughing. As the acute phase subsides, a fibroblastic response develops, resulting in long-term deposition of collagen and fibrosis.[11] Fibrosis leads to reduced tissue viscosity, which dampens the normal vibratory patterns that are required for normal voice.[12] These tissue changes make rehabilitation difficult because there is currently no therapy that can improve the vibratory capacity of the vocal folds.

Because none of the treatment modalities have been clearly shown to help improve postradiation phonation, rehabilitation is often multifaceted, relying on both physician and speech-language pathologists to maximize outcomes. This article serves to first outline important factors in the evaluation of the patient and then discusses both surgical and nonsurgical interventions that may aid rehabilitation.

PATIENT EVALUATION OVERVIEW

Evaluation begins with obtaining a thorough history and physical examination. Aspects of the patient's history that are valuable for guiding treatment include staging of the primary malignancy, treatment course including radiation dose and completion date, response to treatment, antecedent voice concerns or disease, current vocal demand or vocal use, and current vocal concerns.

Many of these aspects can be identified with a review of the medical records from the treating radiation oncologist. A review of the initial staging can help the clinician appreciate the laryngeal subsite (supraglottic, glottic, or subglottic) of the primary tumor and the presence of nodal disease. This information will give the clinician an appreciation for both the anatomic focus of the radiation treatment and the size of the treatment fields if (ie, if radiation was also administered to neck disease). It will also allow the physician to focus their subsequent examinations to survey for recurrence or persistence of disease. A review of the treatment course is helpful to identify the total dose of radiation administered to the larynx and any breaks in treatment that could lead to higher concern for recurrence.

The patient's vocal history should be elicited with a thorough interview before the physical examination. Key portions of the history include preradiation voice changes and whether there was change to the voice throughout RT. The patient's current concerns should also be discussed and can highlight perceived changes in effort or strain of phonation, difficulty with projection, decreased pitch flexibility or loss of range, and breathiness. These concerns are discussed from a subjective perspective but can be quantified with the use of the Voice-Handicap Index (VHI) and the Voice-Related Quality of Life. These are completed by the patient and may be useful to quantify the patients' experience and concerns to follow their progression over time.

Physical examination should include a full head and neck examination along with a thorough laryngeal examination and objective assessment of the quality of the patient's voice. The vocal quality of the patient who has received radiation can vary dramatically from almost no deficits to complete aphonia, and a multidisciplinary approach incorporating physicians and speech-language pathologists should be used to fully assess the patient's voice. For objective assessment of voice quality, either the GRBAS scale (Grade, Roughness, Breathiness, Aesthenia, Strain) or the CAPE-V (The Consensus Auditory-Perceptual Evaluation of Voice) scale can be used in objectifying the subjective perception of a patient's voice. Both are useful for perceptual assessment of a patient's voice but may not necessarily correlate to the patient's self-assessment; however, the GRBAS and CAPE-V scales correlate to each other when graded by experienced speech-language pathologists.[13–16]

Acoustic parameters are another means to obtain objective measures of vocal quality. Parameters measured include fundamental frequency and range, intensity, maximum phonation time, formant patterns, airway pressures, shimmer, jitter, signal-to-noise ratio, and cepstral peak prominence. When compared with patients who do not receive radiation, patients who do receive radiation have decreased intensity, pitch range, and maximum phonation time; they also demonstrate increased shimmer, jitter, and subglottic air pressure.[8–10,17] Cepstral peak prominence is an objective measure that has recently shown strong correlations with other objective voice measures but also perceptual measures of voice changes.[18] It has not been studied specifically in the irradiated larynx and is an area that will require focus for future research.

Visualization of the larynx should also be performed as part of the physical examination. Indirect mirror laryngoscopy can be effective in identifying large lesions of the larynx or vocal fold immobility but is incapable of identifying subtle mucosal lesions or vibratory abnormalities. Indirect transnasal fiberoptic laryngoscopy can be used when the patient's gag reflex limits adequate visualization of the larynx with a mirror. This technique shares similar limitations as mirror laryngoscopy in that the provider may not identify small mucosal lesions or vibratory deficiencies. Indirect videostroboscopic visualization of the larynx is indicated to further examine the vibratory action of the vocal folds and affords the benefits of a magnified examination of the larynx.[19] Whenever possible, recordings of voice samples and laryngeal examination should be archived to compare in future examinations.[20]

Videostroboscopy is an incredible advancement in our ability to visualize subtle vibratory deficits created by RT, but it offers an incomplete visualization of the larynx. Videostroboscopy creates the illusion of vibration by capturing out-of-phase images and merging them together into a fluid video. In doing so, the technique omits segments of laryngeal motion and vibration when the light source is not active. High-speed cinematography captures 2000 to 6000 images per second and, therefore, captures the most images omitted by stroboscopy. Enormous amounts of video data are created for each examination, which can make interpretation and clinical application challenging.[21] Videokymography and kymography are ancillary examinations that developed from high-speed cinematography and offer an assessment of the vocal fold mucosa of one narrow coronal plane of the vocal folds. This method allows the examiner to assess symmetry and amplitude of vibration at the selected point of the glottis. Videokymography is more prevalent of an instrument than kymography, but both techniques enrich the data offered by high-speed cinematography; they both show limited, but increasing, clinical application for laryngeal visualization.[22]

Obtaining a thorough history and physical examination are necessary to help build a care plan tailored to the patient. The physician is only one part of this process, however. We find that a thorough interdisciplinary examination performed in concert with speech-language pathology is integral to furthering the identification of concerning objective and subjective patient concerns. We feel this approach offers the most comprehensive patient evaluation and maximizes the potential benefit of therapy.

MANAGEMENT GOALS

Although rehabilitation of the postradiation voice is important, the clinician must always be cognizant of the risk of persistence or recurrence of disease and the need for continued surveillance for secondary malignancies. Once absence of disease is confirmed through examination or ancillary imaging techniques, the goals of therapy are focused on the concerns of the patient. These can be specifically aimed at objective findings identified in clinical evaluation or subjective measures identified by the patient.

BEHAVIORAL TREATMENT OPTIONS

Behavioral (nonpharmacologic) treatment is the mainstay of rehabilitation for the radiated larynx and can be broken down into indirect voice therapy/vocal hygiene and direct voice therapy.

Vocal hygiene primarily centers on hydration. Laryngeal radiation spares the oral cavity and oropharynx so patients usually do not appreciate dry mouth or salivary changes during or after treatment.[23,24] However, laryngeal salivary tissue is damaged by radiation and can result in laryngeal desiccation that can affect vocal performance.[11,25] There are no published data regarding whether this is an early- or late-phase response to radiation, but our clinical experience indicates that desiccation can occur in either timeframe. Patients should maintain adequate systemic hydration to maximize vocal function during and after radiation treatment. Local hydration using environmental humidification or steam inhalation is also beneficial.

Speech therapy is the main treatment modality used for voice rehabilitation after RT. However, few studies have investigated the role of speech therapy in ameliorating vocal deficits that develop during or after RT. The use of speech therapy was first described in the 1960s as a method to minimize the acute effects of radiation during treatment.[26] Since then, studies have attempted to find short- and long-term benefits from behavioral intervention. van Gogh and colleagues[27] investigated the role of voice therapy after treatment of early glottic carcinoma with a case-control study, but the patient population of the study also included patients who underwent transoral laser resection of disease. They did not identify a difference in voice outcomes (both VHI and acoustic analyses) between the laser endoscopic treatment and radiation treatment but did demonstrate an overall improvement in vocal outcomes with speech therapy. This study did not identify or standardize the exercises performed and it did not report the patient compliance in adopting treatment strategies. A subsequent study prospectively examined the role of voice therapy for patients who received radiation but again did not standardize or describe the methods of voice therapy implemented stating, "the type of voice therapy could be chosen freely according to the patient's needs." This study found improvement of VHI, noise-to-harmonic ratio, jitter, and shimmer after a 12-week therapy regimen; these improvements are sustained up to 1 year after cessation of treatment.[28] Additional research also shows that patients note an increase in loudness despite lack of significant changes to objective acoustic parameters.[29]

A Swedish group formalized an approach to postradiation voice therapy and reported its findings in 2013. The study investigated a 10-week regimen that focused on relaxation, posture, and supported breathing during phonation; the study reported subjective and objective data 1 and 6 months after speech therapy. Patients started treatment 1 month after the conclusion of radiation. This case-control study found improvement of jitter and shimmer in treatment and control groups but also showed improvement in harmonics-to-noise ratio and maximum phonation time in the treatment group. Patients undergoing treatment also showed subjective improvements in vocal fatigue and volume compared with the control cohort.[30] It is, however, important to note this study included 3 patients with T3 disease who are considered outside the realm of discussion for this article.

Our clinical experience is that voice therapy designed to reduce inflammation (with semioccluded vocal tract phonation) and maintain or improve flexibility (with glide exercises) is beneficial for patients who receive radiation and subjectively decreases effort and strain with phonation. Further research is needed to examine the role of speech-language pathology in rehabilitative efforts.

PHARMACOLOGIC TREATMENT OPTIONS

Ideal targets of pharmacologic treatment include minimizing damage to the superficial lamina propria, decreasing laryngeal inflammation, and minimizing fibrosis. As with nonpharmacologic treatments, there are few supporting studies showing benefit to the irradiated larynx.

Currently available treatments focus on decreasing laryngeal inflammation. Injection of steroids has been used in other settings to reduce laryngeal scar and fibrosis, but their application has not been studied specifically in the irradiated larynx.[31] There is evidence for the use of proton pump inhibitors (PPIs) in the setting of laryngeal trauma to optimize epithelial regrowth, but there is no published evidence that the use of PPIs is beneficial in the setting of laryngeal radiation. Despite this, many providers prescribe PPIs empirically for patients undergoing laryngeal RT.[32]

Few pharmacologic treatments have progressed beyond the laboratory, but several investigational treatments may minimize or prevent radiation changes. In vitro models show enhanced remodeling of the lamina propria after injection of tumor necrosis factor alpha (TNF-α) and Carbylan-GSX.[33] Bone marrow–derived mesenchymal stromal cell application has shown promise for increasing matrix metalloproteinase 1, a marker for extracellular matrix remodeling and tissue generation, in in vitro models but has not been applied to in vivo trials.[34]

Further research into pharmaceutical agents is required before definitive recommendations can be applied to rehabilitation of the postradiation larynx.

SURGICAL TREATMENT OPTIONS

Surgical treatments are designed to help restore vibratory capacity or improve laryngeal closure, but the research supporting their use is limited. In an ideal situation, the clinician would be able to replace damaged superficial lamina propria to restore the vibratory capacity of the radiated larynx. To date, proposed treatments involving injection of material into the superficial lamina propria to replicate or improve mucosal pliability have not shown consistent improvements.[31,35,36] Because replacement of the lamina propria is currently not an available treatment option, surgical intervention is limited to 3 main arenas: surgical interventions designed to soften scar, interventions to improve laryngeal configuration for voicing through vocal fold augmentation surgery, and interventions to replace lamina propria through experimental procedures with fat implantation or engineered tissues.

Tissue manipulation for vocal fold scar has 2 main areas of focus. One technique is an attempt at scar excision or redirection. This was initially described with cold instrumentation by Bouchayer and Cornut[37] but has also been adapted for focal scar release with CO_2 laser.[38] However, this has not been described—and may not be applicable—for treatment of diffuse scarring and fibrosis often exhibited in the delayed postradiation larynx. A second treatment strategy involves the use of pulse dye laser (PDL) to increase turnover of the extracellular matrix within the superficial lamina propria. Initial investigations of PDL in treating cutaneous scar showed alteration of collagenase expression, alteration of collagen protein structure, and resultant softening of scar tissue.[39] PDL has been used to treat vocal fold scar and results in increased subjective assessment of posttreatment mucosal pliability and objective improvement of VHI, jitter, and shimmer. However, postradiation scar only accounted for 18% of the study population, and results of the patients who received radiation were not reported separately.[40]

Vocal fold augmentation with injection laryngoplasty or medialization thyroplasty has been used to improve glottic competency and reduce the subglottic pressure required to drive phonation.[12] Importantly, augmentation does not directly address vocal fold scar and does not improve the vibratory capacity of the vocal folds. Research on the effects of vocal fold augmentation in the radiated larynx is also limited, but one study is applicable. Although the aim of their study was not to directly assess the capacity of injection laryngoplasty for rehabilitation of dysphonia secondary to radiation, Chang and colleagues[41] showed that patients undergoing injection laryngoplasty with calcium hydroxylapatite for glottic insufficiency who received radiation have worse vocal improvement than patients who did not receive radiation. Our own clinical experience finds that patients are able to improve the intensity of phonation with injection laryngoplasty, but treatment does little to help the ease and quality of their voice. In our experience, type I thyroplasty has been used but brings the added risks of chondronecrosis and implant extrusion after manipulation of irradiated laryngeal framework. This risk may be dose dependent and is a topic of future investigation.

The Gray minithyrotomy was introduced in 1999 as a treatment of sulcus vocalis and vocal fold scar.[42] This procedure has been applied to patients with radiation-induced scar in 2 studies. The largest series contains 22 patients, of which, 2 had radiation fibrosis.[43] Both patients showed improvement in mucosal wave propagation and glottal competency, but one of the patients had mucosal perforation during their procedure. That patient had undergone a previous procedure to release the scar, but the complication highlights the altered mucosal tissue of the patient who has received radiation. The other study started with 3 patients who received radiation, but only one patient remained in the study to completion. That patient noted improvement in his VHI-10 score and had a self-reported improvement in voice, but did not demonstrated increased mucosal pliability or glottic competency.[44]

The Gray minithyrotomy could be adapted to allow replacement of the superficial lamina propria, but as previously mentioned, an adequate synthetic or engineered substitute is not available. Surgical intervention may become more beneficial with the advancement of tissue engineering, but currently treatment options remain limited.

SUMMARY

The laryngeal changes brought on by RT can be measured with both subjective and objective measures. Unfortunately, our ability to rehabilitate these changes is limited.

There is insufficient data to recommend specific pharmacologic treatments, and the published surgical interventions are not well powered enough to definitively endorse specific intervention. Speech-language pathology currently is the most researched rehabilitation technique and remains the primary means for improving patient's phonation after definitive radiation treatment, but the optimal specific treatment modalities are not clear. Further research is needed to not only improve our rehabilitation potential but also to develop means to prevent or minimize the deleterious effects of radiation during treatment.

REFERENCES

1. Sanguineti G, Ricchetti F, McNutt T, et al. Dosimetric predictors of dysphonia after intensity-modulated radiotherapy for oropharyngeal carcinoma. Clin Oncol 2014; 26:32–8.
2. Epstein BE, Lee DJ, Kashima H, et al. Stage T1 glottic carcinoma: results of radiation therapy or laser excision. Radiology 1990;175:567–70.
3. Jones AS, Fish B, Fenton JE, et al. The treatment of early laryngeal cancers (T1-T2 N0): surgery or irradiation? Head Neck 2004;26(2):127–35.
4. Hintz B, Charyula K, Chandler JR, et al. Randomized study of local control and survical following radical surgery or radiation therapy in oral and laryngeal carcinomas. J Surg Oncol 1979;12:61–74.
5. Chacko DC, Hendrickson FR, Fisher A. Definitive irradiation of T1-T4N0 larynx cancer. Cancer 1983;51(6):994–1000.
6. Aref A, Dworkin J, Devi S, et al. Objective evaluation of the quality of voice following radiation therapy for T1 glottic cancer. Radiother Oncol 1997;45:149–53.
7. Verdonck-de Leeuw IM, Keus RB, Hilgers FJ, et al. Consequences of voice impairment in daily life for patients following radiotherapy for early glottic cancer: voice quality, vocal function, and vocal performance. Int J Radiat Oncol Biol Phys 1999;109:241–8.
8. Verdonck-de Leeuw IM, Hilgers FJ, Keus RB, et al. Multidimensional assessment of voice characteristics after radiotherapy for early glottic cancer. Laryngoscope 1999;109:241–8.
9. Hocevar-Boltezar I, Zargi M. Voice quality after radiation therapy for early glottic cancer. Arch Otolaryngol Head Neck Surg 2000;126(9):1097–100.
10. Lehman JJ, Bless DM, Brandenburg JH. An objective assessment of voice production after radiation therapy for stage I squamous cell carcinoma of the glottis. Otolaryngol Head Neck Surg 1988;98:121–9.
11. Johns MM, Kolachala V, Berg E, et al. Radiation fibrosis of the vocal fold: from man to mouse. Laryngoscope 2012;112:S107–25.
12. Findelhor BK, Titze IR, Durham PL. The effect of viscosity changes in the vocal folds on the range of oscillation. J Voice 1988;1:320–5.
13. Dejonckere PH, Wieneke GH. GRBAS-scaling of pathological voices: reliability, clinical relevance and differentiated correlation with acoustic measurements, especially with cepstral measurements. Proceedings of the 22nd IALP Congress. Hanover (Germany), August 10-14, 1992.
14. Kempster GB, Gerratt BR, Verdolini Abbott K, et al. Consensus auditory-perceptual evaluation of voice: development of a standardized clinical protocol. Am J Speech Lang Pathol 2009;18(2):124–32.
15. Karnell MP, Melton SD, Childes JM, et al. Reliability of clinician-based (GRBAS and CAPE-V) and patient-based (V-RQOL and IPVI) documentation of voice disorders. J Voice 2007;21(5):576–90.

16. Nemr K, Simoes-Zenari M, Cordeiro GF, et al. GRBAS and CAPE-V scales: high reliability and consensus when applied at different times. J Voice 2012;26(6): 812.e17–22.

17. Stoicheff ML. Voice following radiotherapy. Laryngoscope 1975;85(4):608–18.

18. Heman-Ackah YD, Sataloff RT, Laureyns G, et al. Quantifying the cepstral peak prominence, a measure of dysphonia. J Voice 2014;28(6):783–8.

19. Sulica L. Laryngoscopy, stroboscopy and other tools for the evaluation of voice disorders. Otolaryngol Clin North Am 2013;46(1):21–30.

20. Hirano M, Yoshida Y, Yoshida T, et al. Strobofiberscopic video recording of vocal fold vibration. Ann Otol Rhinol Laryngol 1985;94(6):584–7.

21. Patel R, Dailey S, Bless D. Comparison of high-speed digital imaging with stroboscopy for laryngeal imaging of glottal disorders. Ann Otol Rhinol Laryngol 2008; 117:413–24.

22. Qiu Q, Schutte HK. A new generation videokymography for routine clinical vocal fold examination. Laryngoscope 2006;116:85–91.

23. Mendenhall WM, Parsons JT, Buatti JM, et al. Advances in radiotherapy for head and neck cancer. Semin Surg Oncol 1995;11:256–64.

24. Laoufi S, Mirghani H, Janot F, et al. Voice quality after treatment of T1a glottic cancer. Laryngoscope 2014;124(6):1398–401.

25. Hartley NA, Thibeault SL. Systemic hydration: relating science to clinical practice in vocal health. J Voice 2014;28(5):652.e1–20.

26. Fex S, Henriksson B. Phoniatric treatment combined with radiotherapy of laryngeal cancer for the avoidance of radiation damage. Acta Otolaryngol Suppl 1969;263:128–9.

27. van Gogh CD, Verdonck-de Leeuw I, Boon-Kamma BA, et al. The efficacy of voice therapy in patients after treatment for early glottic carcinoma. Cancer 2006;106(1):95–105.

28. van Gogh CD, Verdonck-de Leeuw I, de Bruin MD, et al. Long-term efficacy of voice therapy in patients with voice problems after treatment of early glottic cancer. J Voice 2012;26(3):398–401.

29. Tuomi L, Andrell P, Finizia C. Effects of voice rehabilitation after radiation therapy for laryngeal cancer: a randomized controlled study. Int J Radiat Oncol Biol Phys 2014;89(5):964–72.

30. Tuomi L, Bjorkner E, Finizia C. Voice outcome in patients treated for laryngeal cancer: efficacy of voice rehabilitation. J Voice 2014;28(1):62–8.

31. Mortensen M, Woo P. Office steroid injections of the larynx. Laryngoscope 2006; 116:1735–9.

32. Kantas I, Balatsouras DG, Kamargianis N, et al. The influence of laryngopharyngeal reflux in the healing of laryngeal trauma. Eur Arch Otorhinolaryngol 2009; 266(2):253–9.

33. Chen X, Thibeault SL. Role of Tumor necrosis factor-alpha in wound repair in human vocal fold fibroblasts. Laryngoscope 2010;120:1819–25.

34. Chen X, Thibeault SL. Cell-cell interaction between vocal fold fibroblasts and bone marrow mesenchymal stromal cells in three-dimensional hyaluronan hydrogrel. J Tissue Eng Regen Med 2013. [Epub ahead of print].

35. Ford CN, Bless DM, Loftus JM. Role of injectable collagen in the treatment of glottic insufficiency: a study of 119 patients. Ann Otol Rhinol Laryngol 1992;101: 237–47.

36. Shaw GY, Szewczyk MA, Searle J, et al. Autologous fat injection into the vocal folds: technical considerations and long-term follow-up. Laryngoscope 1997; 107:177–86.

37. Bouchayer M, Cornut G. Microsurgery for benign lesions of the vocal folds. Ear Nose Throat J 1988;67(6):446–56.
38. Martinez Arias A, Remacle M, Lawson G. Treatment of vocal fold scar by carbon dioxide laser and collagen injection: retrospective study on 12 patients. Eur Arch Otorhinolaryngol 2010;267:1409–14.
39. Orringer JS, Hammerberg C, Hamilton T, et al. Molecular effects of photodynamic therapy for photoaging. Arch Dermatol 2008;144:1296–302.
40. Mortensen MM, Woo P, Ivey C, et al. The use of the pulse dye laser in the treatment of vocal fold scar: a preliminary study. Laryngoscope 2008;118(10):1884–8.
41. Chang J, Courey MS, Al-Jurf SA, et al. Injection Laryngoplasty Outcomes in Irradiated and nonirradiated unilateral vocal fold paralysis. Laryngoscope 2014;124:1895–9.
42. Gray SD, Bielamowicz SA, Titze IR, et al. Experimental approaches to vocal fold alteration; introduction to the minithyrotomy. Ann Otol Rhinol Laryngol 1999;108:1–9.
43. Paniello RC, Sulica L, Khosla SM, et al. Clinical experience with Gray's Mini-thyrotomy procedure. Ann Otol Rhinol Laryngol 2008;117:437–42.
44. Mallur PS, Gartner-Schmidt J, Rosen CA. Voice outcomes following the gray mini-thyrotomy. Ann Otol Rhinol Laryngol 2012;121(7):490–6.

Contemporary Surgical Management of Early Glottic Cancer

Dana M. Hartl, MD, PhD[a],*, Daniel F. Brasnu, MD[b]

KEYWORDS

- Larynx • Glottis • Squamous cell carcinoma • Transoral laser surgery
- Conservation laryngeal surgery • Organ preservation

KEY POINTS

- Transoral laser microsurgery (TLM) is the main surgical treatment modality for T1-T2 glottic squamous cell carcinoma.
- The European Laryngological Society classifications for transoral laser resection should be used to describe the extent of TLM resection.
- Thyroid cartilage invasion is rare and T2 tumors with decreased vocal fold mobility have a higher risk for occult cartilage invasion.
- Local control rates are lower for T1 lesions with tumors infiltrating the anterior commissure and for T2 lesions with decreased vocal fold motion, whether treated with TLM or open surgery.
- For tumors staged cN0, no prophylactic treatment of the neck is currently recommended.

INTRODUCTION

Early glottic squamous cell carcinoma—Tis, T1a, T1b, and T2[1]—carries a relatively good prognosis, whether treated surgically or nonsurgically with radiation therapy (RT). Epidemiologically, these tumors continue to be related to tobacco consumption and only exceptionally to human papillomavirus infection compared with oropharyngeal cancers.[2] Surveillance, Epidemiology, and End Results data from the United States show that the incidence of laryngeal cancer has been decreasing by an average

The authors have nothing to disclose.
[a] Department of Head and Neck Oncology, Institut de Cancérologie Gustave Roussy, 114 rue Edouard Vaillant, Villejuif 94805, France; [b] Otolaryngology Head & Neck Surgery, University Hospital Cancer Pole, Paris Descartes University and Sorbonne Paris III University, Hôpital Européen Georges Pompidou, 20, rue Leblanc, Paris Cedex 15 75908, France
* Corresponding author.
E-mail address: dana.hartl@gustaveroussy.fr

of 2.5% per year in the twenty-first century, with decreasing death rates (http://seer. cancer.gov/statfacts/html/laryn.html).

The main goal of conservation surgery is to optimize local control to avoid total laryngectomy. With optimum local control, overall survival is related to N stage, metastases, second primaries, and comorbidity. Due to the generally favorable outcomes of T1-T2 glottic tumors treated with different modalities, morbidity, voice quality, quality of life, and cost are issues to be considered when choosing a treatment modality for these early-stage tumors. This article covers the oncologic results related to surgical management of early glottic cancer, with voice quality covered in an article by Hartl DM and colleagues elsewhere in this issue.

PATIENT EVALUATION

The clinical and radiologic work-up for patients with glottic cancer is discussed in an article elsewhere in this issue. Particular attention should be given, however, to the evaluation of vocal fold mobility—normal, diminished, or fixed—due to the prognostic significance of this factor and the influence it may have on the surgical (or nonsurgical) treatment choice.[3,4] Vocal fold mobility may be decreased (and the tumor classified then as T2) due to a bulky tumor but also due to paraglottic space invasion or invasion of the cricoarytenoid joint.[5] Imaging is required to determine these deeper tumor extensions. These early-stage tumors have a low rate of thyroid cartilage invasion, but tumors with decreased vocal fold mobility have a higher risk of occult cartilage invasion.[6] Laryngeal tumors are amenable to conservation surgery if the tumor can be resected with free margins (R0) while conserving 2 essential entities:

- The functional integrity of the cricoid cartilage must be intact, keeping in mind that resection of the anterior arch is possible without destabilizing the cricoid ring. An unstable cricoid cartilage leads to laryngeal stenosis and permanent tracheostomy. The cricoid ring is the only complete cartilaginous ring in the airway and must be preserved in conservation surgery to prevent postoperative stenosis. Cricoid cartilage invasion is always a contraindication to conservation laryngeal surgery due to the impossibility of obtaining sufficient margins while maintaining a patent airway postoperatively.[7] Tumors with anterior subglottic extension sparing the upper edge of the cricoid cartilage can be treated with conservation laryngeal surgery, and anterior subglottic extension up to, but not invading, the cricoid cartilage may be amenable to supracricoid partial laryngectomy with tracheohyoidoepiglottopexy (discussed later). Posteriorly, the cricoid cartilage is situated closely below the level of the vocal folds (a few millimeters), so that posterior tumors reaching the upper border of the cricoid cartilage are generally a contraindication to conservation laryngeal surgery.
- At least 1 cricoarytenoid unit, comprised of the cricoid, an arytenoid cartilage, the cricoarytenoid joint and muscles, and the corresponding recurrent laryngeal nerve, must be preserved to preserve the sphincteric function of the larynx during swallowing, to avoid aspiration that can lead to pneumonia and death. The sphincteric function of the larynx (or neolarynx) also serves as the voice generator, with the mucosa generating sound waves.

Individual patients must also meet certain requirements for conservation laryngeal surgery, be it by transoral resection or open surgery. Comorbidities and tolerance of general anesthesia must be evaluated. Pulmonary function testing is recommended if open surgery or extended resection (arytenoid) is planned, and the risk of postoperative aspiration requires that patients have sufficient pulmonary reserve to withstand this possible complication in the immediate postoperative period. Procedures having little effect on the sphincteric function of the larynx, such as cordectomy, are of low risk in the elderly whereas a hemilaryngectomy or a supracricoid partial laryngectomy alters the sphincteric function of the larynx and, therefore, is considered a high-risk procedure in elderly patients.[8] Conservation surgery has been performed for malignant and benign laryngeal tumors in children for whom the same oncologic and functional principles apply.[9,10] Voice considerations and patient preferences should be discussed as well and are addressed in another article of this issue.

In historical series of T1-T2 glottic tumors treated with small-field RT without prophylactic treatment of the neck, reported rates of nodal recurrence were approximately 4%.[11,12] In surgical series, the rate of occult neck metastases for early glottic cancer was less than 10%.[13-15] It is now generally agreed that prophylactic treatment of the neck is not necessary if the tumor is classified radiologically as cN0.

TRANSORAL LASER MICROSURGERY

The carbon dioxide laser beam with a wavelength of 10,600 nm is absorbed by water, limiting the depth of extension in human tissues and thus allowing cutting precision without widespread thermal damage to surrounding tissues. Transoral laser resection via suspension microlaryngoscopy was first developed in the 1970s by Strong and Jako,[16] with the first laser cordectomy reported in 1975. Extension of the technique to include resection of laryngeal structures other than the vocal fold was promoted by Eckel and Thumfart,[17] Rudert,[18] Steiner and Ambroch,[19] and otherss in the 1980s and widespread use of the technique appeared in the 1990s. In the past 25 years, TLM has largely supplanted open conservation laryngeal surgery, with pioneers of the technique showing early on that complete, oncologically sound resection is possible transorally with low morbidity and without diminished oncologic outcomes.[20-25] Technological advances in laryngeal microscopy and lasers have facilitated access to this type of surgery, which is now considered the gold standard for treatment of early glottic cancer.[26]

Transoral laser resection is based on à la carte resection, after tumor spread and sparing noninvolved structures, contrary to other techniques in which resection follows anatomic landmarks rather than following the tumor itself. In most cases, tracheotomy is not required, simplifying the postoperative course. Limits to the technique include patients whose morphology limits exposure of the larynx transorally and short neck, small oral aperture, large tongue base, retrognathism, and/or tooth mobility or dental prosthetic work in the anterior maxillary region. Exposure of the larynx may be facilitated by resection of the false vocal fold (vestibulectomy) and/or by partial resection of the epiglottis, particularly the petiole of the epiglottis for exposure of the anterior commissure.

Today the European Laryngological Society classification for transoral laser resection of glottic cancers is largely used.[27,28] It takes into account depth of resection in the vocalis muscle and extent of resection, including the anterior commissure and supraglottic and subglottic structures (particularly suited to T2 lesions). **Table 1** summarizes this classification.

Resection Margins

A resection margin of 2 mm is sufficient in glottic cancer, as opposed to other cancer sites in the head and neck.[29-31] On histopathologic examination, positive or close margins (<2 mm) may be observed, sometimes only due to loss of tissue peripheral to the tumor due to thermocoagulation artifacts and/or shrinkage of the specimen when

Table 1
The European Laryngological Society classification for transoral laser microsurgical resection of glottic tumors

Classification	Description	Schematic Representation
Type I	Subepithelial	
Type II	Subligamental	
Type III	Transmuscular	
Type IV	Total cordectomy	
Type Va	Extension to the anterior commissure	—
Type Vb	Extension to the arytenoid cartilage	
Type Vc	Extension to the false vocal fold	

(continued on next page)

Table 1 (continued)		
Classification	Description	Schematic Representation
Type Vd	Extension to the subglottis	
Type VI	Anterior commissure and petiole of the epiglottis	

Data from Remacle M, Eckel HE, Antonelli A, et al. Endoscopic cordectomy. A proposal for a classification by the Working Committee, European Laryngological Society. Eur Arch Otorhinolaryngol 2000;257(4):227–31. Figures from Remacle M, Van Haverbeke C, Eckel H, et al. Proposal for revision of the European Laryngological Society classification of endoscopic cordectomies. Eur Arch Otorhinolaryngol 2007;264(5):499–504; with permission and La chirurgie conservatrice des cancers du larynx et du pharynx: Les monographies Amplifon, n° 39. Paris: Amplifon, 2005; with permission.

fixated for pathology. The significance of positive or close margins has been the subject of several retrospective studies with conflicting results: some studies found a significant increase in local recurrence for patients with close or positive margins[32,33] whereas others were not able to show a significant difference.[4,34–36] Deep positive margins, however, after the first TLM resection contributed to lower local control and organ preservation rates for Peretti and colleagues.[4] Thus, close superficial margins may undergo complementary resection with the laser or a close watch-and-wait follow-up. Patients with positive margins at the first operation may benefit from a second-look procedure. A systematic second look in cases of free margins is not necessary, however. To limit the risk of positive margins, some teams use frozen section analysis, with high predictive values.[33,37] Patients should always be informed preoperatively as to the risk of a second look procedure.

Local Control and Organ Preservation

Reported local control rates for Tis to T2 range from 80% to 100%. Reported ultimate laryngeal preservation rates (taking into account radiation or surgery for salvage) for Tis range from 85% to 100%, for T1 carcinoma from 89% to 100%, and for T2 carcinoma from 83% to 100%.[3,17,23,38–40] A major advantage in TLM is that is leaves all options open for treating recurrences: repeat TLM, RT, or open surgery. In all of the reported series, even those only including T1a treated with transoral or open resection, there is a small but constant percentage of patients (1%–2%) who suffer from recurrence not amenable to organ preservation and who require a total laryngectomy.[35,41] There do not seem to be any detectable risk factors enabling pretreatment selection of these patients, but advances in understanding of tumor biology may one day enable foreseeing this type of evolution and treat these selected patients accordingly.

For tumors classified as Tis, initial local control ranges from 56% to 100%. These superficial lesions may arise in the form of glottic field cancerization and local recurrences after TLM may be adjacent to the area initially resected or at some distance or even on the other vocal fold. This may also explain the high rate of recurrence after vocal fold stripping, which has largely been supplanted by the type I cordectomy.[42] Repeat TLM is often successful in case of local recurrence.

Anterior Commissure

The anterior commissure tendon (Broyles ligament) is generally a barrier to spread of early glottic cancer. Even with this relative barrier, anterior commissure cancers may spread upward toward the petiole of the epiglottis and downward in the subglottic region and invade the cricothyroid membrane. At the inferior border of the thyroid cartilage, these tumors may even extend upward along the thyroid cartilage deep to the outer layer of the perichondrium.[5,43,44] Furthermore, in many cases, the cartilage at the anterior commissure is ossified; anatomically there is no perichondrium at this level and Broyles ligament may be ruptured, making the anterior commissure a weak spot for tumor infiltration.[45,46] Tumors involving the anterior commissure generally have a higher risk of local recurrence after TLM, be they Tis, T1a, T1b, or T2.[47–56] For infiltrating, particularly ulcerating, tumors, the higher recurrence rate is possibly due to deep superior and inferior extensions along the inner perichodrium of the thyroid cartilage, with microscopic spreading to the preepiglottic space and/or to the subglottis but also possibly to microscopic cartilage invasion at this weak spot in the cartilage.[45] Thyroid cartilage resection may be warranted for these tumors. Resection of the anterior commissure with TLM (type Va or VI cordectomies) can lead to the formation of an anterior glottic web, which negatively affects voice. Several investigators have reported a decreased incidence in web formation with the intraoperative application of mitomycin C[57,58] or with the use of cryotherapy just after the laser resection.[59]

Tumors classified as T2 with posterior extension tend to have lower local control rates with transoral laser resection.[60] Tumors extending into Morgagni ventricle and supraglottic extension of glottic carcinoma (transglottic carcinoma) have a higher risk of thyroid cartilage invasion, especially for anteriorly or posteriorly extending tumors.[43] Transoral resection must take these potential tumor extensions into account with resection as needed of the inner thyroid perichondrium, thyroid cartilage, or arytenoid cartilage. T2 tumors with deep extension into the paraglottic space (classified as pT3) not initially detected on preoperative imaging, have also been shown to have lower local control and organ preservation rates using TLM alone.[3]

Complications of Transoral Laser Microsurgery

For Tis, T1, and T2 glottic cancers, the rate of minor complications with no lasting side effects has been reported as less than 5%, and major complications—in particular secondary hemorrhage, dyspnea, and severe aspiration pneumonia—are rare (less than 2%).[19,61–63] The complication rate for glottic lesions is lower than that of supraglottic and hypopharyngeal tumors due to a higher risk of hemorrhage, aspiration, and edema after resection of these tumors. For glottic tumors, the risk of a complication is related to the extent of surgery (related to tumors size),[61] with a higher rate of aspiration particularly for extended cordectomies with arytenoid resection. Local infection with perichondritis was reported in 1 of the 109 cases of glottic tumors reported by

Vilaseca-Gonzalez and colleagues[61] due to wide endolaryngeal exposure of the thyroid cartilage. The infection resolved after 3 weeks of antibiotics with spontaneous laryngeal re-epithelialization. Subcutaneous emphysema is also a rare occurrence and was related to resection of the cricothyroid membrane, in this same cohort. Again, the emphysema resolved spontaneously in a few days without further complication. In this same series, pneumonia occurred in 2% of cases and 1 case of postoperative dyspnea occurred. Thus, the rate of tracheostomy is less than 1% for these tumors. Oral intake is allowed generally on day 1 or 2 and hospital stay is 1 to 4 days.[58] For early glottic carcinoma, the rate of complications seems comparable between elderly (>75 years of age) and nonelderly patients.[64]

ROBOT-ASSISTED TRANSORAL LARYNGEAL SURGERY

The width of the robotic arms and difficulty with triangulation in the limited laryngeal space are main factors contributing to the slow take-off of robot-assisted transoral surgery for early glottic cancer, the supraglottic larynx being more accessible with the surgical robot in its current configuration.[65] Exposure of the larynx may be facilitated with tongue retraction and partial epiglottectomy.[66,67] Another limiting factor, until recently, was the degree of thermal injury inflicted on the glottis by the monopolar cautery used with robotic surgery. Recently, this problem has been addressed by the development of a CO_2 laser fiber, which decreases the depth and width of thermal dissemination to adjacent tissues.[68,69] The role of robotic assistance for early glottic cancer remains to be fully explored.[70] The considerations of this transoral resection are the same as those for TLM, mainly the significance of close or positive margins, anterior commissure involvement, and outcomes for tumors with decreased vocal fold mobility or deep paraglottic invasion.

OPEN SURGERY

Open conservation laryngeal surgery (partial laryngectomy) is performed less and less for early glottic cancer particularly due to the accessibility of TLM and its comparable oncologic outcomes, with much lower morbidity.[26] The use of nonsurgical organ preservation with RT or chemoradiation has also contributed to the decline in open surgery. Contemporary knowledge of tumor extensions and modern imaging techniques have also contributed to the decline in open surgery for these early tumors: the low rate of thyroid cartilage invasion in particular makes wide cartilage resections most often unnecessary for these early tumors.[6]

Many different techniques have been described for open resection of T1-T2 glottic cancer, which can be globally classified into vertical partial laryngectomies—entailing a vertical thyrotomy, with open cordectomy, frontolateral vertical partial laryngectomy, vertical hemilaryngectomies, and frontal anterior vertical partial laryngectomy—and horizontal partial laryngectomies, essentially represented by the family of supracricoid partial laryngectomies with cricohyoidoepiglottopexy, cricohyoidopexy, or tracheocricohyoidoepiglottopexy.[7]

Open cordectomy and the frontolateral vertical laryngectomy are the open equivalents of the type IV and type Va endoscopic resections (see **Table 1**). Neither technique requires a tracheostomy,[71] but, as for TLM, the complete resection of the vocalis muscle is a major factor in voice quality (see article elsewhere in this issue for details). TLM allows tailoring of the resection to the depth of invasion of the tumor, which open surgery does not. Initial local control for T1a glottic tumors treated with these techniques ranges from 90% to 100% and is comparable to TLM.[24] With these open procedures, swallowing should be monitored closely, because some patients may have temporary low-grade clinical aspiration (in particular elderly patients). Speech and oral feeding can start on postoperative day 1. Subcutaneous emphysema can develop and can be managed conservatively by reopening the wound and replacing a nonsuction drain, with or without a compression dressing. Laryngeal granuloma is rarely obstructive and usually heals spontaneously or with oral steroid treatment. A further issue with these 2 types of open procedures—as with TLM in the region of the anterior commissure—is anterior glottic web formation, another factor influencing voice quality. A reconstruction procedure, pulling the false vocal fold down to cover the cartilage defect (a false vocal fold flap) has been described and shown to decrease granuloma and web formation in open frontolateral partial laryngectomies.[72]

Vertical hemilaryngectomy is essentially an equivalent of a type Vc TLM resection associated with resection of part of the thyroid cartilage. The standard vertical partial laryngectomy or standard hemilaryngectomy entails resection of the entire vocal fold, the entire ventricle and false vocal fold, part of the thyroid ala, and the vocal process of the arytenoid cartilage. It is generally indicated for T2 glottic tumors with normal or impaired vocal fold mobility. Resection of the thyroid ala allows more extensive resection of the paraglottic space for tumors with deep muscular invasion, but the posterior part of the paraglottic space lateral to the arytenoid is not resected with this technique. Extended hemilaryngectomies involve the same resection as the standard hemilaryngectomy but also if necessary entail resection of the ipsilateral arytenoid with disarticulation and/or resection of the entire anterior commissure.

The frontal anterior laryngectomy[73] corresponds to an extended type VI resection with TLM but including thyroid cartilage resection. It remains an excellent indication for glottic carcinoma with extension to the anterior commissure, due to the wide cartilaginous resection that this technique provides at this level, the simple postoperative course, and the satisfactory voice quality. This technique does not address tumor extension superiorly to the preepiglottic space, however, which is resected in the supracricoid procedures.

Supracricoid partial laryngectomies allow total removal of the thyroid cartilage for excellent control of anterior commissure and ventricular tumors. The entire paraglottic space is removed bilaterally. One arytenoid cartilage can be removed, allowing for resection of glottic and supraglottic tumors extending posteriorly. The major portion of the preepiglottic space, excluding the lateral horns, can be safely resected. The entire cricothyroid membrane and anterior subglottis are resected. The preservation of the epiglottis (supracricoid partial laryngectomy with cricohyoidoepiglottopexy) is determined by the proximity of the tumor to the petiole of the epiglottis and the extension to the preepiglottic space.[8]

For these extensive resections, the restrictions to conservation laryngeal surgery for glottic cancer—a stable cricoid and a functional cricoarytenoid unit—apply to all the different techniques, keeping in mind that for resections extending beyond cordectomy or frontolateral partial laryngectomy, some aspiration is expected postoperatively. Thus, pulmonary function should be normal. Patients with chronic respiratory insufficiency or decreased pulmonary reserve should not undergo this type of surgery. Heart disease, uncontrolled severe diabetes, or other severe comorbidities and age greater than 70 are relative contraindications to extended vertical and supracricoid partial laryngectomies as well.[74,75]

Local control with open surgery for T1 carcinomas ranges from 90% to 100% and for T2 from 69% to 100%. Comparing historical cohorts, for T2 tumors, supracricoid partial laryngectomies seem to provide higher rates of local control and laryngeal preservation than vertical hemilaryngectomies (69%–78% for hemilaryngectomies vs 83%–100% for supracricoid laryngectomies), particularly for T2 tumors with decreased vocal fold mobility.[7,76] This is most likely due to the lack of resection of the posterior paraglottic space in a classic vertical hemilaryngectomy, which is addressed by supracricoid resections, but also possibly to a higher rate of occult thyroid cartilage invasion, which may be missed by radiologic assessment.[77]

The postoperative course after open conservation laryngeal surgery (except cordectomy and frontolateral partial laryngectomy) is complex, requiring management of the tracheostomy and feeding tube. Hospitalization is 1 to 3 weeks on average, whereas for TLM it is less than 1 to 2 days. Recovery of efficient swallowing is long, particularly after supracricoid partial laryngectomies, with 42% of patients still demonstrating clinical aspiration after 1 month but 97% recovering swallowing without aspiration at 1 year.[78,79] In large published series by specialized centers, the rate of permanent gastrostomy was 2% to 3%, permanent tracheostomy less than 1%, and total laryngectomy for intractable aspiration 2%.[8] The advantage of open surgery is to allow more extensive resection for more extensive tumors, with epiglottoplasty or cricohyodopexies to reconstruct a functional larynx, in terms of both swallowing and voice.

EVALUATION OF OUTCOME

There currently are no data with high-level evidence (randomized controlled trial) directly comparing the oncologic outcomes of surgery with RT or chemoradiation for T1-T2 glottic carcinoma. One small prospective randomized study, however, was recently published, with the main objective to compare voice quality between TLM and RT, with 32 patients in the TLM group and 28 patients in the RT group.[80] The local control rate at 2 years was the same in both groups.

Three meta-analyses have compared oncologic data for early glottic cancer treated with these 2 modalities. Higgins and colleagues[81] in 2009 included 26 studies and found no difference in local control or organ preservation. The data suggested improved overall survival for patients treated with TLM (odds ratio 1.48; 95% CI, 1.19–1.85). This finding, however, may be related to biases inherent in the retrospective studies included, favoring RT for patients with comorbidities that could influence survival. The meta-analysis published by Feng and colleagues[82] in 2011 included 5 studies reporting local control rates of T1-T2 glottic cancer and found no significant difference between the treatment modalities. Finally, Abdurehim and colleagues[83] included 10 studies in their meta-analysis of oncologic outcomes for T1a glottic cancer and found no difference between TLM and RT with regard to local control, disease-specific survival, or overall survival. Thus, for Tis, T1, and T2 glottic carcinoma, there is currently no evidence showing a difference in local control, disease-specific survival, or organ preservation for either surgery or RT.

Retrospective studies have shown that T2 tumors with decreased vocal fold mobility have a higher risk of recurrence compared with T2 tumors with normal laryngeal mobility, whether treated with surgery or RT, with supracricoid partial laryngectomies providing the highest rate of local control, at the cost of extensive open surgery with a long postoperative course.[7,77]

The bulk of the current literature (low-level evidence) shows that tumors involving the anterior commissure, whether Tis, T1, or T2, have a higher risk of recurrence than tumors not involving the anterior commissure. Reported rates of local control and laryngeal preservation range from 75% to 98% for T1 tumors involving the anterior commissure, with comparable results reported with TLM, open surgery, and RT. For T1b tumors involving the anterior commissure, a recent retrospective cohort study found no difference in oncologic outcomes between RT and TLM.[84]

Three previous retrospective studies, however, found that initial local control and final laryngeal preservation were higher with surgery versus RT for T1-T2 tumors involving the anterior commissure.[54,85,86] This tends to favor surgery in this scenario, although other factors need to be taken into consideration.

Many other factors should be taken into account when offering treatment of T1-T2 glottic carcinoma. Patient age is a major factor. Elderly patients are at risk for major complications, such as aspiration pneumonia and death, after open partial laryngectomies extending beyond the confines of the vocal fold. Extended TLM, particularly to the arytenoid region, may also put these patients at risk for major aspiration. Pulmonary and cardiovascular comorbidities and illnesses affecting wound healing and infection must also be factored in. Younger patients are at risk for second primary cancers and for late complications of RT, such as fibrosis and chondronecrosis, which may appear decades later. Finally, RT can only be performed once, and failures often require salvage total laryngectomy. Thus for Tis and T1a tumors, it has been suggested (even by radiation oncologists) that RT be saved for situations in which all surgical options have failed, particularly in young patients.[87–89]

Cost and duration of treatment may be important issues for some patients or in some health care settings. Several studies have calculated that the cost of RT outweighs that of TLM.[90–93] RT generally requires 5 to 7 weeks, and accessibility of treatment centers may make this option unrealistic. Finally, voice issues, discussed in a separate article in this issue, need to be discussed with the patient. The decision should always be made in a multidisciplinary setting, providing patients with as much loyal information and guidance as possible.

SUMMARY

For early-stage glottic squamous cell carcinoma T1-T2, TLM is the main surgical modality today, with rates of local control and laryngeal preservation ranging from 85% to 100% and low morbidity. For extensive lesions, in particular ulcerating anterior commissure lesions or T2 lesions with decreased vocal fold mobility or posterior extensions, open conservation laryngeal surgery may enable wider resections than TLM but at costs of a longer hospital stay and higher postoperative morbidity. Surgery provides results that are comparable to nonsurgical treatment options (RT and concurrent chemoradiation), while reserving RT for recurrences or second primary cancers, particularly in younger patients.

REFERENCES

1. Sobin LH, Gospodarowicz MK, Wittekind CW. TNM classification of malignant tumors. In: Cancer UIUA, editor. 7th edition. West Sussex (United Kingdom): Wiley-Blackwell; 2010. p. 39–45.
2. Si-Mohamed A, Badoual C, Hans S, et al. An unusual human papillomavirus type 82 detection in laryngeal squamous cell carcinoma: case report and review of literature. J Clin Virol 2012;54(2):190–3.
3. Peretti G, Piazza C, Mensi MC, et al. Endoscopic treatment of cT2 glottic carcinoma: prognostic impact of different pT subcategories. Ann Otol Rhinol Laryngol 2005;114(8):579–86.
4. Peretti G, Piazza C, Cocco D, et al. Transoral CO(2) laser treatment for T(is)-T(3) glottic cancer: the University of Brescia experience on 595 patients. Head Neck 2010;32(8):977–83.
5. Kirchner JA. Growth and spread of laryngeal cancer as related to partial laryngectomy. Can J Otolaryngol 1974;3(4):460–8.

6. Hartl DM, Landry G, Hans S, et al. Organ preservation surgery for laryngeal squamous cell carcinoma: low incidence of thyroid cartilage invasion. Laryngoscope 2010;120(6):1173–6.

7. Hartl D, Brasnu D, Fried M. Conservation surgery for glottic cancer. In: Fried MP, Ferlito A, editors. The larynx. 3rd edition. San Diego (CA): Plural Publishing; 2009. p. 515–43.

8. Brasnu DF. Supracricoid partial laryngectomy with cricohyoidopexy in the management of laryngeal carcinoma. World J Surg 2003;27(7):817–23.

9. Goyal P, Kellman RM. Frontolateral hemilaryngectomy for the management of a case of pediatric squamous cell carcinoma of the larynx. Laryngoscope 2005; 115(6):965–7.

10. Hartl DM, Roger G, Denoyelle F, et al. Extensive lymphangioma presenting with upper airway obstruction. Arch Otolaryngol Head Neck Surg 2000;126(11): 1378–82.

11. Smee R, Bridger GP, Williams J, et al. Early glottic carcinoma: results of treatment by radiotherapy. Australas Radiol 2000;44(1):53–9.

12. Chera BS, Amdur RJ, Morris CG, et al. T1N0 to T2N0 squamous cell carcinoma of the glottic larynx treated with definitive radiotherapy. Int J Radiat Oncol Biol Phys 2010;78(2):461–6.

13. Erdag TK, Guneri EA, Avincsal O, et al. Is elective neck dissection necessary for the surgical management of T2N0 glottic carcinoma? Auris Nasus Larynx 2013; 40(1):85–8.

14. Coskun HH, Medina JE, Robbins KT, et al. Current philosophy in the surgical management of neck metastases for head and neck squamous cell carcinoma. Head Neck 2014;37(6):915–26.

15. Psychogios G, Mantsopoulos K, Bohr C, et al. Incidence of occult cervical metastasis in head and neck carcinomas: development over time. J Surg Oncol 2013; 107(4):384–7.

16. Strong MS, Jako GJ. Laser surgery in the larynx. Early clinical experience with continuous CO_2 laser. Ann Otol Rhinol Laryngol 1972;81(6):791–8.

17. Eckel HE, Thumfart WF. Laser surgery for the treatment of larynx carcinomas: indications, techniques, and preliminary results. Ann Otol Rhinol Laryngol 1992; 101(2 Pt 1):113–8.

18. Rudert H. Experiences with the CO2 laser with special reference to the therapy of vocal cord carcinoma. Laryngol Rhinol Otol 1983;62(11):493–8 [in German].

19. Steiner W, Ambroch P. Endoscopic laser surgery of the upper aerodigestive tract. Stuttgart (Germany): Thieme; 2000.

20. Canis M, Ihler F, Martin A, et al. Transoral laser microsurgery for T1a glottic cancer: Review of 404 cases. Head Neck 2014;37(6):889–95.

21. Canis M, Martin A, Ihler F, et al. Transoral laser microsurgery in treatment of pT2 and pT3 glottic laryngeal squamous cell carcinoma - results of 391 patients. Head Neck 2014;36(6):859–66.

22. Ambrosch P. The role of laser microsurgery in the treatment of laryngeal cancer. Curr Opin Otolaryngol Head Neck Surg 2007;15(2):82–8.

23. Davis RK. Endoscopic surgical management of glottic laryngeal cancer. Otolaryngol Clin North Am 1997;30(1):79–86.

24. Hartl DM, Ferlito A, Brasnu DF, et al. Evidence-based review of treatment options for patients with glottic cancer. Head Neck 2011;33(11):1638–48.

25. Suarez C, Rodrigo JP, Silver CE, et al. Laser surgery for early to moderately advanced glottic, supraglottic, and hypopharyngeal cancers. Head Neck 2012; 34(7):1028–35.

26. Silver CE, Beitler JJ, Shaha AR, et al. Current trends in initial management of laryngeal cancer: the declining use of open surgery. Eur Arch Otorhinolaryngol 2009;266(9):1333–52.

27. Remacle M, Eckel HE, Antonelli A, et al. Endoscopic cordectomy. A proposal for a classification by the Working Committee, European Laryngological Society. Eur Arch Otorhinolaryngol 2000;257(4):227–31.

28. Remacle M, Van Haverbeke C, Eckel H, et al. Proposal for revision of the European Laryngological Society classification of endoscopic cordectomies. Eur Arch Otorhinolaryngol 2007;264(5):499–504.

29. Ossoff RH, Sisson GA, Shapshay SM. Endoscopic management of selected early vocal cord carcinoma. Ann Otol Rhinol Laryngol 1985;94(6 Pt 1):560–4.

30. Lam KH, Lau WF, Wei WI. Tumor clearance at resection margins in total laryngectomy. A clinicopathologic study. Cancer 1988;61(11):2260–72.

31. Lee JG. Detection of residual carcinoma of the oral cavity, oropharynx, hypopharynx, and larynx: a study of surgical margins. Trans Am Acad Ophthalmol Otolaryngol 1974;78(1):ORL49–53.

32. Ansarin M, Santoro L, Cattaneo A, et al. Laser surgery for early glottic cancer: impact of margin status on local control and organ preservation. Arch Otolaryngol Head Neck Surg 2009;135(4):385–90.

33. Remacle M, Matar N, Delos M, et al. Is frozen section reliable in transoral CO(2) laser-assisted cordectomies? Eur Arch Otorhinolaryngol 2010;267(3):397–400.

34. Michel J, Fakhry N, Duflo S, et al. Prognostic value of the status of resection margins after endoscopic laser cordectomy for T1a glottic carcinoma. Eur Ann Otorhinolaryngol Head Neck Dis 2011;128(6):297–300.

35. Hartl DM, de Mones E, Hans S, et al. Treatment of early-stage glottic cancer by transoral laser resection. Ann Otol Rhinol Laryngol 2007;116(11):832–6.

36. Sigston E, de Mones E, Babin E, et al. Early-stage glottic cancer: oncological results and margins in laser cordectomy. Arch Otolaryngol Head Neck Surg 2006; 132(2):147–52.

37. Fang TJ, Courey MS, Liao CT, et al. Frozen margin analysis as a prognosis predictor in early glottic cancer by laser cordectomy. Laryngoscope 2013;123(6): 1490–5.

38. Ambrosch P, Kron M, Steiner W. Carbon dioxide laser microsurgery for early supraglottic carcinoma. Ann Otol Rhinol Laryngol 1998;107(8):680–8.

39. Koufman JA. The endoscopic management of early squamous carcinoma of the vocal cord with the carbon dioxide surgical laser: clinical experience and a proposed subclassification. Otolaryngol Head Neck Surg 1986;95(5):531–7.

40. Peretti G, Nicolai P, Piazza C, et al. Oncological results of endoscopic resections of Tis and T1 glottic carcinomas by carbon dioxide laser. Ann Otol Rhinol Laryngol 2001;110(9):820–6.

41. Kerr P, Mark Taylor S, Rigby M, et al. Oncologic and voice outcomes after treatment of early glottic cancer: transoral laser microsurgery versus radiotherapy. J Otolaryngol Head Neck Surg 2012;41(6):381–8.

42. Nguyen C, Naghibzadeh B, Black MJ, et al. Carcinoma in situ of the glottic larynx: excision or irradiation? Head Neck 1996;18(3):225–8.

43. Kirchner JA. Growth and spread of laryngeal cancer as related to partial laryngectomy. Laryngoscope 1975;85(9):1516–21.

44. Kirchner JA. Invasion of the framework by laryngeal cancer. Surgical and radiological implications. Acta Otolaryngol 1984;97(5–6):392–7.

45. Kirchner JA, Fischer JJ. Anterior commissure cancer–a clinical and laboratory study of 39 cases. Can J Otolaryngol 1975;4(4):637–43.

46. Nakayama M, Brandenburg JH. Clinical underestimation of laryngeal cancer. Predictive indicators. Arch Otolaryngol Head Neck Surg 1993;119(9):950–7.

47. Hakeem AH, Tubachi J, Pradhan SA. Significance of anterior commissure involvement in early glottic squamous cell carcinoma treated with trans-oral CO2 laser microsurgery. Laryngoscope 2013;123(8):1912–7.

48. Pearson BW, Salassa JR. Transoral laser microresection for cancer of the larynx involving the anterior commissure. Laryngoscope 2003;113(7):1104–12.

49. Steiner W, Ambrosch P, Rodel RM, et al. Impact of anterior commissure involvement on local control of early glottic carcinoma treated by laser microresection. Laryngoscope 2004;114(8):1485–91.

50. Sachse F, Stoll W, Rudack C. Evaluation of treatment results with regard to initial anterior commissure involvement in early glottic carcinoma treated by external partial surgery or transoral laser microresection. Head Neck 2009;31(4):531–7.

51. Chone CT, Yonehara E, Martins JE, et al. Importance of anterior commissure in recurrence of early glottic cancer after laser endoscopic resection. Arch Otolaryngol Head Neck Surg 2007;133(9):882–7.

52. Bradley PJ, Rinaldo A, Suarez C, et al. Primary treatment of the anterior vocal commissure squamous carcinoma. Eur Arch Otorhinolaryngol 2006;263(10):879–88.

53. Rucci L, Bocciolini C, Romagnoli P, et al. Risk factors and prognosis of anterior commissure versus posterior commissure T1-T2 glottic cancer. Ann Otol Rhinol Laryngol 2003;112(3):223–9.

54. Zohar Y, Rahima M, Shvili Y, et al. The controversial treatment of anterior commissure carcinoma of the larynx. Laryngoscope 1992;102(1):69–72.

55. Zohar Y, Strauss M. Laser surgery for vocal cord carcinoma involving the anterior commissure. Ann Otol Rhinol Laryngol 1989;98(10):836–7.

56. Szyfter W, Leszczynska M, Wierzbicka M, et al. Value of open horizontal glottectomy in the treatment for T1b glottic cancer with anterior commissure involvement. Head Neck 2013;35(12):1738–44.

57. Roh JL, Yoon YH. Prevention of anterior glottic stenosis after bilateral vocal fold stripping with mitomycin C. Arch Otolaryngol Head Neck Surg 2005;131(8):690–5.

58. Roh JL, Yoon YH. Prevention of anterior glottic stenosis after transoral microresection of glottic lesions involving the anterior commissure with mitomycin C. Laryngoscope 2005;115(6):1055–9.

59. Knott PD, Milstein CF, Hicks DM, et al. Vocal outcomes after laser resection of early-stage glottic cancer with adjuvant cryotherapy. Arch Otolaryngol Head Neck Surg 2006;132(11):1226–30.

60. Davis RK, Hadley K, Smith ME. Endoscopic vertical partial laryngectomy. Laryngoscope 2004;114(2):236–40.

61. Vilaseca-Gonzalez I, Bernal-Sprekelsen M, Blanch-Alejandro JL, et al. Complications in transoral CO2 laser surgery for carcinoma of the larynx and hypopharynx. Head Neck 2003;25(5):382–8.

62. Rudert HH, Werner JA. Endoscopic resections of glottic and supraglottic carcinomas with the CO2 laser. Eur Arch Otorhinolaryngol 1995;252(3):146–8.

63. Peretti G, Nicolai P, Redaelli De Zinis LO, et al. Endoscopic CO2 laser excision for tis, T1, and T2 glottic carcinomas: cure rate and prognostic factors. Otolaryngol Head Neck Surg 2000;123(1 Pt 1):124–31.

64. Sesterhenn AM, Dunne AA, Werner JA. Complications after CO(2) laser surgery of laryngeal cancer in the elderly. Acta Otolaryngol 2006;126(5):530–5.

65. Smith RV. Transoral robotic surgery for larynx cancer. Otolaryngol Clin North Am 2014;47(3):379–95.

66. De Virgilio A, Park YM, Kim WS, et al. How to optimize laryngeal and hypopharyngeal exposure in transoral robotic surgery. Auris Nasus Larynx 2013;40(3):312–9.
67. Vicini C, Leone CA, Montevecchi F, et al. Successful application of transoral robotic surgery in failures of traditional transoral laser microsurgery: critical considerations. ORL J Otorhinolaryngol Relat Spec 2014;76(2):98–104.
68. Blanco RG, Ha PK, Califano JA, et al. Transoral robotic surgery of the vocal cord. J Laparoendosc Adv Surg Tech A 2011;21(2):157–9.
69. Remacle M, Matar N, Lawson G, et al. Combining a new CO2 laser wave guide with transoral robotic surgery: a feasibility study on four patients with malignant tumors. Eur Arch Otorhinolaryngol 2012;269(7):1833–7.
70. Lallemant B, Chambon G, Garrel R, et al. Transoral robotic surgery for the treatment of T1-T2 carcinoma of the larynx: preliminary study. Laryngoscope 2013; 123(10):2485–90.
71. Brumund KT, Gutierrez-Fonseca R, Garcia D, et al. Frontolateral vertical partial laryngectomy without tracheotomy for invasive squamous cell carcinoma of the true vocal cord: a 25-year experience. Ann Otol Rhinol Laryngol 2005;114(4): 314–22.
72. Biacabe B, Crevier-Buchman L, Hans S, et al. Phonatory mechanisms after vertical partial laryngectomy with glottic reconstruction by false vocal fold flap. Ann Otol Rhinol Laryngol 2001;110(10):935–40.
73. Sedlacek K. Reconstructive anterior and lateral laryngectomy with the use of the epiglottis for the pedicle graft. Cesk Otolaryngol 1965;14(6):328–34 [in Czech].
74. Naudo P, Laccourreye O, Weinstein G, et al. Complications and functional outcome after supracricoid partial laryngectomy with cricohyoidoepiglottopexy. Otolaryngol Head Neck Surg 1998;118(1):124–9.
75. Naudo P, Laccourreye O, Weinstein G, et al. Functional outcome and prognosis factors after supracricoid partial laryngectomy with cricohyoidopexy. Ann Otol Rhinol Laryngol 1997;106(4):291–6.
76. Laccourreye O, Laccourreye L, Garcia D, et al. Vertical partial laryngectomy versus supracricoid partial laryngectomy for selected carcinomas of the true vocal cord classified as T2N0. Ann Otol Rhinol Laryngol 2000;109(10 Pt 1): 965–71.
77. Hartl DM. Evidence-based practice: management of glottic cancer. Otolaryngol Clin North Am 2012;45(5):1143–61.
78. Laccourreye H, Laccourreye O, Weinstein G, et al. Supracricoid laryngectomy with cricohyoidopexy: a partial laryngeal procedure for selected supraglottic and transglottic carcinomas. Laryngoscope 1990;100(7):735–41.
79. Laccourreye H, Laccourreye O, Weinstein G, et al. Supracricoid laryngectomy with cricohyoidoepiglottopexy: a partial laryngeal procedure for glottic carcinoma. Ann Otol Rhinol Laryngol 1990;99(6 Pt 1):421–6.
80. Aaltonen LM, Rautiainen N, Sellman J, et al. Voice quality after treatment of early vocal cord cancer: a randomized trial comparing laser surgery with radiation therapy. Int J Radiat Oncol Biol Phys 2014;90(2):255–60.
81. Higgins KM, Shah MD, Ogaick MJ, et al. Treatment of early-stage glottic cancer: meta-analysis comparison of laser excision versus radiotherapy. J Otolaryngol Head Neck Surg 2009;38(6):603–12.
82. Feng Y, Wang B, Wen S. Laser surgery versus radiotherapy for T1-T2N0 glottic cancer: a meta-analysis. ORL J Otorhinolaryngol Relat Spec 2011;73(6):336–42.
83. Abdurehim Y, Hua Z, Yasin Y, et al. Transoral laser surgery versus radiotherapy: systematic review and meta-analysis for treatment options of T1a glottic cancer. Head Neck 2012;34(1):23–33.

84. Taylor SM, Kerr P, Fung K, et al. Treatment of T1b glottic SCC: laser vs. radiation–a Canadian multicenter study. J Otolaryngol Head Neck Surg 2013;42:22.
85. Rucci L, Gallo O, Fini-Storchi O. Glottic cancer involving anterior commissure: surgery vs radiotherapy. Head Neck 1991;13(5):403–10.
86. Bron LP, Soldati D, Zouhair A, et al. Treatment of early stage squamous-cell carcinoma of the glottic larynx: endoscopic surgery or cricohyoidoepiglottopexy versus radiotherapy. Head Neck 2001;23(10):823–9.
87. Fein DA, Mendenhall WM, Parsons JT, et al. T1-T2 squamous cell carcinoma of the glottic larynx treated with radiotherapy: a multivariate analysis of variables potentially influencing local control. Int J Radiat Oncol Biol Phys 1993;25(4): 605–11.
88. Holland JM, Arsanjani A, Liem BJ, et al. Second malignancies in early stage laryngeal carcinoma patients treated with radiotherapy. J Laryngol Otol 2002; 116(3):190–3.
89. Burns JA, Har-El G, Shapshay S, et al. Endoscopic laser resection of laryngeal cancer: is it oncologically safe? Position statement from the American Broncho-Esophagological Association. Ann Otol Rhinol Laryngol 2009;118(6):399–404.
90. Smith JC, Johnson JT, Cognetti DM, et al. Quality of life, functional outcome, and costs of early glottic cancer. Laryngoscope 2003;113(1):68–76.
91. Goor KM, Peeters AJ, Mahieu HF, et al. Cordectomy by CO2 laser or radiotherapy for small T1a glottic carcinomas: costs, local control, survival, quality of life, and voice quality. Head Neck 2007;29(2):128–36.
92. Cragle SP, Brandenburg JH. Laser cordectomy or radiotherapy: cure rates, communication, and cost. Otolaryngol Head Neck Surg 1993;108(6):648–54.
93. Sjogren EV, van Rossum MA, Langeveld TP, et al. Voice outcome in T1a midcord glottic carcinoma: laser surgery vs radiotherapy. Arch Otolaryngol Head Neck Surg 2008;134(9):965–72.

Voice Outcomes of Transoral Laser Microsurgery of the Larynx

Dana M. Hartl, MD, PhD[a],*, Samia Laoufi, MD[b],
Daniel F. Brasnu, MD[c]

KEYWORDS

- Larynx • Glottis • Cancer • Voice • Laser • Surgery

KEY POINTS

- Voice results seem to stabilize after 6 months, and analysis of definitive voice results should not be performed before 6 and 12 months after transoral laser microsurgery.
- Almost-normal voice, measured both subjectively and objectively, can be expected in most patients after type I, II, or III cordectomies, but voice outcomes are unpredictable for a given patient.
- Voice outcomes are particularly related to the glottal gap on phonation, which itself is related to the depth of resection of the vocalis muscle and the extent of cordectomy beyond the vocal fold.
- No direct, prospective comparison of transoral laser microsurgery with radiation therapy for comparable tumors (depth and extent) has ever been performed.
- Meta-analyses of retrospective studies comparing transoral laser microsurgery with radiation therapy have only found small or no differences in voice quality, and the only currently published randomized study (with only 60 patients) found more breathiness and impact of hoarseness on daily life in the transoral laser microsurgery group.

INTRODUCTION

Transoral laser microsurgery (TLM) has become the mainstay in the surgical treatment of early-stage (TisT1T2) glottic cancer with excellent oncologic outcomes, comparable to nonsurgical options (**Table 1**). When evaluating different treatment options for early glottic cancer, factors such as patient age and comorbidities, treatment availability,

The authors have nothing to disclose.
[a] Service Rhône, Department of Head and Neck Oncology, Institut de Cancérologie Gustave Roussy, 114 rue Edouard Vaillant, Villejuif 94805, France; [b] Department of Head and Neck Oncology, Institut de Cancérologie Gustave Roussy, 114 rue Edouard Vaillant, Villejuif 94805, France; [c] Otolaryngology-Head and Neck Surgery, University Hospital Cancer Specialities Pole, University Paris Descartes and Sorbonne Nouvelle, Hôpital Européen Georges Pompidou, 20, rue Leblanc, Paris 75908 Cedex 15, France
* Corresponding author.
E-mail address: dana.hartl@gustaveroussy.fr

Otolaryngol Clin N Am 48 (2015) 627–637
http://dx.doi.org/10.1016/j.otc.2015.04.008
0030-6665/15/$ – see front matter © 2015 Elsevier Inc. All rights reserved.

Abbreviations	
GRBAS	Grade Roughness Breathiness Asthenia Strain
RT	Radiation therapy
TLM	Transoral laser microsurgery

cost and duration, and risk of second primary cancer should be taken into consideration. However, because of the favorable prognosis of these tumors, long-term voice quality and quality of life for these patients is the major factor in selecting the type of treatment.

The approach to evaluating the dysphonic patient is described in another article by S. Dailey and colleagues in this issue. This article covers the current literature regarding subjective voice quality and voice-related quality of life and studies with objective acoustic and aerodynamic results after treatment of early glottic cancer with TLM.

WHEN TO EVALUATE VOICE AFTER TRANSORAL LASER MICROSURGERY

The thermal effects of TLM with postoperative inflammation and localized edema generally subside within 1 to 2 months and lead to the formation of scar tissue that can evolve over time. This inflammation and scarring can lead to variable voice quality during the first few months postoperatively. Definitive voice evaluation should be undertaken only when the voice quality has stabilized. Several studies attempted to ascertain the appropriate time after which the voice is stable and thus definitive voice quality is evaluable.

In a prospective cohort study, voices of 106 male patients with T1 tumors treated with type II subligamental cordectomy[1] were recorded preoperatively, then at 3, 6, 12 and 24 months postoperatively. The objective acoustic measurements of jitter, shimmer, and normalized noise energy returned to within the normal range after just 3 months, but the voice fundamental frequency remained in a higher range than normal (140 Hz) even after 24 months.[2]

In a smaller and more heterogeneous study, prospectively evaluating patients preoperatively and at 1, 3, 6, and 12 months, Chu and colleagues[3] found that the

Table 1
Factors affecting voice outcomes after TLM for early (T1–T2) glottic carcinoma

Tumor/Surgery-Related Factors	Healing/Compensation-Related Factors	Patient-Related Factors
Depth of extent of resection • Vocal ligament • Vocalis (thyro-arytenoid) muscle Extent of resection of vocalis muscle in the sagittal plane Resection of the anterior commissure Extended resections to arytenoid, supraglottic, and subglottic structures Type of cordectomy: types I and II vs type III vs types IV, V, and VI	Time lapse after surgery (< 12 mo vs >12 mo) Anterior web formation Compensatory mechanisms to glottal gap • Supraglottic compensation • Crico-thyroid muscle activity	Younger patients vs older patients Voice use, voice professionals Voice expectations Patient's psychological reaction to the diagnosis of cancer

subjective evaluation (grade, roughness, breathiness, asthenia, and strain [GRBAS scale]) and the objective acoustic and aerodynamic parameters improved and then stabilized at 6 months for limited and more extensive resections. In a prospective cohort study, Lester and colleagues[4] found that for the 19 T1 tumors treated with TLM, acoustic and aerodynamic measurements were abnormal 3 months postoperatively but returned to preoperative values after 12 months. Other studies have shown voice stabilization after 12 months.[5,6]

Finally, Spielmann and colleagues,[7] published a systematic review in 2010 encompassing 15 studies comparing voice outcomes in patients treated with TLM versus RT. The authors cite 1 study evaluating voice after 3 months, 3 studies with evaluations after a minimum of 6 months, and the 11 remaining studies evaluating voice after 12 to 24 months or more.

It appears, then, from the literature, that definitive voice evaluation should not be performed before 6 months postoperatively and that it may be more appropriate to evaluate voice after an interval of 12 months because of some heterogeneity in the healing process, possibly affected by the extent of TLM.

Interestingly, in a self-oscillating physical model of the vocal folds, Mendelsohn and colleagues[8] found that adding a scar to the model of the vibrating vocal fold, voice was improved compared with the model of vocal fold resection without scarring. Thus, in real life, it is possible that a certain rigidity of the vocal fold, obtained only after a period of healing, will affect the definitive vocal outcome, either by an acoustic or an aerodynamic mechanism.

HOW IS VOICE SUBJECTIVELY AFTER TRANSORAL LASER MICROSURGERY?

Subjective voice results have been studied in numerous publications of prospective and retrospective cohorts. The methods of subjective evaluation vary among publications, with patient self-reporting or blinded or nonblinded expert reporting. The scales vary from visual analog scales to the GRBAS scale, the most largely used.[9] Many of these publications have been retained in 4 meta-analyses and 1 systematic review.[7,10–13] Only one recent prospective, randomized study comparing voice results after TLM with voice after RT has been published.[14]

In a cross-sectional study of 42 consecutive male patients, evaluated 6 to 48 months postoperatively, Vilaseca and colleagues[15] found that definitive subjective voice quality was correlated to the amount of tissue resected, that is, to the type of cordectomy performed. After a type I cordectomy, two-thirds of patients had a "normal to near-normal" voice, as rated by the otolaryngologist, and, after types II and III, 55% of patients had a normal or near-normal voice, whereas only 25% had a normal or near-normal voice after a type V cordectomy. Thirty-one percent of these latter patients were judged to have severe dysphonia. Compared with normal controls, all of the GRBAS categories, as judged by a speech therapist, were significantly worse after TLM, and particularly for the grade, breathiness, and asthenia categories. On a scale from 0 to 3, type I, II, and III cordectomies resulted in GRBAS scores of approximately 1, whereas more extended cordectomies resulted in GRBAS scores of greater than 2.

Physiologically, a near-normal voice after a type I cordectomy may be explained by the preservation of the superficial lamina propria (Reinke's space), which preserves the mucosal wave, once the mucosa has healed. Deeper cordectomies, however, remove the superficial lamina propria at the tumor site. When the mucosa regenerates, the scar tissue is fixed to the underlying tissues with little or no vibratory qualities.

Similarly, Aaltonen and colleagues,[14] in a prospective study of 32 patients 2 years after TLM, found a median GRBAS score of 1.5. Nineteen percent of their patients had a G score of 0, whereas 7% had a G score of 3. Resection of the anterior portion of the vocal fold was correlated with worse vocal outcomes in this study. Several other studies found the same correlation between the extent of the cordectomy (types V and VI) and a worse subjective vocal outcome.[3,16,17] For exclusively T1a lesions treated with TLM, Czecior and colleagues[18] found that 54% of patients had a G score of 0 to 1, 78% an R score of 0 to 1, 96% a B score of 0 to 1, 99% an A score of 0 to 1, and 58% an S score of 0 to 1. Compared with preoperative voice, Aaltonen and colleagues[14] found a significant improvement in average self-reported hoarseness on a visual analog scale of 0 to 100 after 6 months (50/100 vs 59/100 preoperatively), improving further after 12 months (43/100). Thus, most patients will have normal to near-normal voices after TLM, particularly after type I, II, and III cordectomies. Poorer subjective voice quality is to be expected with more extended cordectomies.

HOW IS VOICE-RELATED QUALITY OF LIFE AFTER TRANSORAL LASER MICROSURGERY?

Some voice-related quality of life studies include studies based on responses to general questions such as "effect of voice on daily living" measured with visual analog scales or Likert scales, but the most widely used metric for evaluating the daily handicap associated with voice quality is the Voice Handicap Index (VHI), either in its initial 30-question version, or its reduced 10-question version. The questionnaire evaluates physical, functional, and emotional domains of voice handicap. Reported scores on the VHI-30, where 120 represents the worst most incapacitating voice, range from 11.5 to 29.2 for T1a glottic cancers treated with TLM.[13,19–24] For comparison, the average VHI in the case of benign vocal fold lesions is approximately 26; for spasmodic dysphonia treated with botulinum toxin it is 22 and after medialization thyroplasty the score is 28.[19] As for subjective voice analysis, the degree of voice handicap is correlated to the depth and extent of the cordectomy. Peretti and colleagues[21] found an average VHI of 6 for superficial type I and II resections, 16.5 for deeper (type III) resections, and 15.8 for type IV or V resections. Roh and colleagues[25] observed the same difference and demonstrated that VHI was also worse if the anterior commissure was resected. Thus, patients generally report low levels of voice handicap after TLM with scores comparable or better than voice handicap after treatment for benign laryngeal diseases.

General quality-of-life questions and questionnaires are also used to evaluate patients with early glottic cancer treated with TLM. On a 0 to 100 visual analog scale of patient self-reported impact on everyday life, Aaltonen and colleagues[14] found scores of 31/100 at 6 months and 32/100 at 12 months. Using a Washington University quality-of-life questionnaire and the short version of the Short Form-12, Vilaseca and colleagues[26] were able to show that overall quality of life was close to normal on average (1139 of a total score of 1200 for the Washington University questionnaire) for T1 or T2 glottic cancers, with normal scores in all of the domains except speech. At 1 year, 69% of the patients in their group of glottic and supraglottic cancers had normal Short Form scores, with supraglottic tumors, radiation therapy (RT) and neck dissection having a negative impact on quality of life. The same group found that "negative changes in daily life" were more frequently observed in younger patients than in older patients. Roh and colleagues[25] compared the speech and social contact domains of the European Organisation for Research and Treatment of Cancer head and neck specific module (EORTC QLQ H&N-35) between superficial and deeper glottic resections and found significantly better scores for type I and II cordectomies versus types III and IV. Thus, again, general quality of life seems to be related to the extent of resection and to patient age, but the impact is minimal to moderate at most.

WHAT ARE THE OBJECTIVE ACOUSTIC RESULTS AFTER TRANSORAL LASER MICROSURGERY?

Many different objective, computer-based acoustic measurements of voice outcomes have been published, with measures of fundamental frequency, pitch variability–related measurements, intensity variability–related measurements, and measurements of the noise component in the acoustic voice recording. Results are often difficult to compare among studies because of the absence of standardization of measurements, the wide range of values that can be considered in the normal range, a significant intra- and interindividual variability in these measurements, and the various computer programs used.[27] In the 8 studies retained for the meta-analysis published by Abdurehim and colleagues,[10] in the TLM groups, jitter ranged from 0.74 ± 1 to 8.67 ± 2.63, and shimmer from 1.31 ± .25 to 13.4 ± 1. In most publications of acoustic analysis, a jitter value of less than 1% and a shimmer value of less than 3.8% are considered normal, and beyond these values voice may be considered pathologic.[28] However, as stated above, there are several different algorithms for detecting the periodicity of fundamental frequency and amplitude and for calculating relative frequency and amplitude perturbations so that reported values may vary according to the computer program used.[27,29] The conditions in which voice is analyzed and recorded—the type of vowel and the duration of the sustained vowel, the type of microphone and recording devices, and surrounding noise—may also influence the results.

In general, however, to cite the work published by Vilaseca and colleagues,[15] "the larger the resection, the higher the number of parameters presenting significant differences with the control group." In this study, voices of 42 consecutive male patients treated with TLM for Tis T1a or T1b cancers were evaluated a minimum of 6 months postoperatively and compared with voices of an age-matched group of 21 male patients. For all types of cordectomy, fundamental frequency increased to an average of 160 Hz, compared with 130 Hz for the control group. Jitter also increased from 1.5 on average to 2.7. Shimmer increased from 0.8 to 1.6 for type V cordectomies. There was no difference in acoustic results according to age (>65 or <65 years) or T stage. Other studies have also found an increase in fundamental frequency after TLM.[2,10,30] In the study by Lester and colleagues,[4] however, compared with preoperative voice with the tumor still in place, acoustic values after TLM were not found to be significantly different. The physiologic basis for the increase in fundamental frequency after TLM is currently unknown. It is possible that the vibrations of the rigid scar band increase fundamental frequency; a decrease of disappearance of the glottic waveform on videostroboscopy has been found after TLM and may contribute to this phenomenon.[7] The observed increase in mean flow rate after TLM with an increase in subglottic pressure may also increase fundamental frequency (see later discussion).[31] Another possible explanation is an increase in cricothyroid muscle activity as compensation for the glottal gap resulting from TLM in analogy to the "paralytic falsetto" observed in vocal fold paralysis.[32]

In dysphonic voices with a low degree of periodicity and a large noise component, automated pitch tracking measurements such as jitter and shimmer may be unreliable, the algorithms having been developed for normal voices with a high degree of periodicity in the acoustic signal.[27,28] Other types of acoustic analyses, less widely studied, aim at characterizing the harmonic structure of voice, for example, and may be more adapted to measuring modifications in abnormal voices. Recently, for example, Stone and colleagues[33] studied cepstral peak prominence in patients treated with TLM for early glottic cancer and found that, despite near-normal measures of jitter and shimmer, the cepstral peak amplitudes were below the normal range, showing perturbation in the harmonic structure of the voice. They, as others, suggest that cepstral analysis, or other acoustic measurement, may be more reliable for characterizing and following acoustic voice quality in patients with abnormal voices.[34,35] This finding is the subject of ongoing research. In any case, acoustic measurements after TLM vary widely but fall within the normal range for many patients, particularly after more superficial resections.[2,15]

WHAT ARE THE OBJECTIVE AERODYNAMIC RESULTS AFTER TRANSORAL LASER MICROSURGERY?

Few studies focus on phonatory aerodynamic measures, with the maximum phonation time and mean phonatory flow rate being reported most often. Most of the studies reporting these measurements show a decrease in maximum phonation time and an increase in mean flow rate after TLM, despite the normal to near-normal subjective and acoustic results in many patients.[3,4,15,16,31] These measurements are most probably the aerodynamic result of the oval closure and incomplete glottal closure observed on videostroboscopy by Aaltonen and colleagues[14] in patients 2 years after TLM. The mean flow rate particularly increased after type V cordectomy in the study by Vilaseca and colleagues,[15] again showing that voice outcomes are related to the extent of resection. Maximum phonation time 1 year after TLM is found to be shorter than preoperative values (tumor in place), again, most probably an aerodynamic effect of the glottal gap resulting from TLM.[4] Zeitels and colleagues[31] found that almost all of the patients in their study had a decrease in vocal efficiency (the ratio of sound pressure level to subglottic pressure) and an increase in subglottic pressure after TLM. They found an improvement in these measures and in voice quality after medialization procedures, which improve "aerodynamic glottal competency" and voice outcomes.

WHAT ARE THE FACTORS INVOLVED IN VOICE QUALITY AFTER TRANSORAL LASER MICROSURGERY?

As shown above, the depth of TLM resection of the vocalis muscle (correlated to the depth of tumor invasion) and the extent of cordectomy are the main factors in voice outcomes after TLM.[16,21,25] Deep extensions to the inner thyroid perichondrium (type IV cordectomy) and extended resections, including the contralateral vocal fold, the arytenoid cartilage, or the false vocal fold (types V) negatively affect voice outcomes.[13] In most patients, voice is normal or near normal after type I or II cordectomies. Type III cordectomy may provide normal to near-normal voice,[4] but the depth of muscle resection in a type III cordectomy varies according to the depth of the tumor, and with deep excisions a type III cordectomy may induce lasting dysphonia. The extent of vocalis muscle resection in the sagittal plane for type III cordectomy has also been found to affect voice outcomes. In one study, a modified type III cordectomy leaving the inferior portion of the vocalis muscle intact provided comparable oncologic results but better results in terms of the GRBAS subjective evaluation, voice handicap index, jitter, shimmer, harmonics-to-noise ratio, and maximum phonation time, most probably because of a higher rate of complete glottic closure visualized postoperatively, with less glottic gap.[36]

It seems from the literature that most studies find that anterior commissure resection results in a worse voice than cordectomy without anterior commissure resection.[17,25,37] This may be caused by, in part, the formation of an anterior glottic scar web in some cases[38] but also by an increased anterior glottal gap compared with less extensive cordectomies. Some studies, however, found that voice was normal to near normal after anterior commissure resection.[39,40] Again, the depth of resection may explain this discrepancy, with superficial resections of the anterior commissure providing normal to near-normal voice, whereas deeper resection may alter voice more significantly. Staged resection is suggested to minimize the risk of anterior web formation.[41] The application of mitomycin C or cryotherapy intraoperatively after resection of anterior commissure tumors may also reduce granuloma and web formation.[42,43]

No study has specifically evaluated voice outcomes in patients requiring a "second-look" procedure (repeat TLM to ascertain margin status), but the study by Stone and colleagues[33] found a correlation between the number of TLM procedures and worse acoustic voice results. Repeat TLM resection may indeed increase the ultimate amount of tissue resected at the glottis and produce further scar tissue.

As seen above, the resulting glottal gap after TLM is a main factor in voice quality. Postsurgical glottal insufficiency can lead to supraglottic compensation with ventricular fold medialization and vibration of supraglottic structures (type II muscle tension dysphonia or MTD) or with compensation at the level of the arytenoids and epiglottis (MTD types III and IV).[4] This phenomenon has been observed after TLM,[4] as after open cordectomies.[44]

In terms of voice handicap and quality of life, the patient's vocal expectations, age, employment, voice use, and the patient's reaction to the diagnosis of cancer are all factors that contribute to widely differing outcomes among patients, despite similar tumors and resection techniques. Even for superficial resections, voice may not be 100% normal after TLM (or after radiation, see later discussion).

HOW DOES VOICE AFTER TRANSORAL LASER MICROSURGERY COMPARE WITH VOICE AFTER RADIATION THERAPY?

Most of the current data comparing voice after TLM with voice after RT for TisT1T2 glottic carcinoma derive at best from retrospective studies of contemporary cohorts, with only one recently published small prospective randomized trial comparing outcomes between these with therapeutic modalities.[14] In addition, 4 meta-analyses and one systematic review have been published in an attempt to obtain enough data (and statistical power) to draw definitive conclusions as to voice outcomes.[7,10–13]

The only currently published prospective, randomized study directly comparing voice outcomes between TLM and RT for early glottic cancer included 60 patients, 31 in the TLM group and 25 in the RT group, all treated for T1a glottic carcinoma.[14] At 2 years posttreatment, patient-rated "hoarseness" did not differ between the 2 groups (43/100 vs 35/100 on a visual analog scale of 0–100) but "impact on everyday life" was significantly higher in the TLM group (32/11 vs 8/100). On an expert-rated GRBAS scale, patients with tumor at the anterior portion of the vocal fold (6 patients of 31) had significantly higher scores of breathiness than the RT group (1.52 vs .28), but no difference in GRBAS scores was found for tumors located in the mid- or posterior portions of the vocal fold. Videostroboscopy showed a significantly higher proportion of patients with an irregular, oval, or incomplete glottic closure on phonation in the TLM group. Thus, it would seem that in some respects, voice outcome was more favorable for the RT group, but, as seen above, the poorer outcome was related particularly to TLM in anterior vocal fold lesions and less to midfold lesions.

A recent meta-analysis included 19 studies with 858 patients in the TLM group and 871 in the RT group.[10] Only 11 studies contained data on functional outcome, however, with significant heterogeneity. No statistically significant differences were found in maximum phonation time (55 patients in the TLM vs 57 patients in the RT group), jitter, or shimmer (including 6 studies with approximately 100 patients in each group) or VHI (including 4 studies with 125 patients TLM group and 96 in the RT group).

An earlier meta-analysis included 9 studies with voice outcomes and found a slight superiority of RT for maximum phonation time, fundamental frequency, phonation intensity range, and GRBAS versus a slight superiority of TLM for jitter and shimmer.[11] The authors made it clear that the cohort sizes were small, even after pooling all of the studies, and that treatment and evaluation were heterogeneous among the studies, including some patients with speech therapy, often heterogeneous follow-up time, and nonblinded voice evaluations.

The meta-analysis of VHI outcomes by Cohen and colleagues[13] included 6 studies with only T1 glottic carcinoma: 202 patients in the TLM group and 91 patients in the RT group. There was no significant difference in VHI, although the time of VHI evaluation in the studies was either unreported or 3, 6, or 12 postoperative months. Feng and colleagues[12] were unable to perform a meta-analysis of the 6 trials that they had retained for VHI evaluation because of too much heterogeneity.

Finally, in a systematic review of 15 studies, Spielmann and colleagues[7] found more studies reporting higher scores of voice handicap (VHI-10) in patients treated with TLM versus RT, but the range of scores on VHI-10 was 9.5 to 12 (vs 3.5–8 in the RT group), reflecting only a mild voice handicap.[45]

Thus, most currently published data show that TLM and RT provide comparable results in terms of voice outcomes and voice-related quality of life. The small differences between these 2 treatment modalities in some studies most probably reflect that these studies, even the only prospective randomized study published, did not include comparable tumors in terms of depth and extent in both treatment groups. A truly randomized trial with sufficient statistical power comparing TLM and RT needs to evaluate depth of tumor infiltration of the vocalis muscle and the extent of the tumor along and beyond the vocal fold and randomly assign patients according to these tumor characteristics, which, as we have seen, are the main factors in ultimate voice outcomes.

SUMMARY

Voice outcomes after TLM are determined by the depth and extent of tissue resection, which are dictated by the depth of tumor invasion and tumor extensions. The depth and extent of resection determine the extent of scar and anterior web formation and the degree of glottal insufficiency. The pathophysiology of compensatory mechanisms such as hyperfunctional activity is currently poorly understood. Thus, for a given patient, the exact voice outcome is unpredictable, and even for a type I cordectomy, voice may not return to normal postoperatively. From a subjective or acoustic viewpoint, for type I cordectomies, one can expect a normal or near-normal voice in up to two-thirds of patients and for type II or III cordectomies a normal to near-normal voice in 50% or more of cases. However, voice handicap is low in most cases and overall quality of life is normal. Automated pitch tracking acoustic measurements (jitter and shimmer) may not be optimal for evaluating voice quality after TLM, and studies of other types of acoustic measurements (eg, spectrum based) are warranted. Studies comparing TLM with RT have not been able to demonstrate significant differences in voice outcomes with any high-level evidence, and few have taken into account voice-related tumor factors such as tumor depth and extent.

REFERENCES

1. Remacle M, Eckel HE, Antonelli A, et al. Endoscopic cordectomy. A proposal for a classification by the Working Committee, European Laryngological Society. Eur Arch Otorhinolaryngol 2000;257(4):227–31.

2. van Gogh CD, Verdonck-de Leeuw IM, Wedler-Peeters J, et al. Prospective evaluation of voice outcome during the first two years in male patients treated by radiotherapy or laser surgery for T1a glottic carcinoma. Eur Arch Otorhinolaryngol 2012;269(6):1647–52.

3. Chu PY, Hsu YB, Lee TL, et al. Longitudinal analysis of voice quality in patients with early glottic cancer after transoral laser microsurgery. Head Neck 2012; 34(9):1294–8.

4. Lester SE, Rigby MH, MacLean M, et al. 'How does that sound?': objective and subjective voice outcomes following CO(2) laser resection for early glottic cancer. J Laryngol Otol 2011;125(12):1251–5.

5. List MA, Ritter-Sterr CA, Baker TM, et al. Longitudinal assessment of quality of life in laryngeal cancer patients. Head Neck 1996;18(1):1–10.

6. Hammerlid E, Silander E, Hornestam L, et al. Health-related quality of life three years after diagnosis of head and neck cancer–a longitudinal study. Head Neck 2001;23(2):113–25.

7. Spielmann PM, Majumdar S, Morton RP. Quality of life and functional outcomes in the management of early glottic carcinoma: a systematic review of studies comparing radiotherapy and transoral laser microsurgery. Clin Otolaryngol 2010;35(5):373–82.

8. Mendelsohn AH, Xuan Y, Zhang Z. Voice outcomes following laser cordectomy for early glottic cancer: a physical model investigation. Laryngoscope 2014; 124(8):1882–6.

9. Hirano M, Hirade Y, Kawasaki H. Vocal function following carbon dioxide laser surgery for glottic carcinoma. Ann Otol Rhinol Laryngol 1985;94(3):232–5.

10. Abdurehim Y, Hua Z, Yasin Y, et al. Transoral laser surgery versus radiotherapy: systematic review and meta-analysis for treatment options of T1a glottic cancer. Head Neck 2012;34(1):23–33.

11. Higgins KM, Shah MD, Ogaick MJ, et al. Treatment of early-stage glottic cancer: meta-analysis comparison of laser excision versus radiotherapy. J Otolaryngol Head Neck Surg 2009;38(6):603–12.

12. Feng Y, Wang B, Wen S. Laser surgery versus radiotherapy for T1-T2N0 glottic cancer: a meta-analysis. ORL J Otorhinolaryngol Relat Spec 2011;73(6):336–42.

13. Cohen SM, Garrett CG, Dupont WD, et al. Voice-related quality of life in T1 glottic cancer: irradiation versus endoscopic excision. Ann Otol Rhinol Laryngol 2006; 115(8):581–6.

14. Aaltonen LM, Rautiainen N, Sellman J, et al. Voice quality after treatment of early vocal cord cancer: a randomized trial comparing laser surgery with radiation therapy. Int J Radiat Oncol Biol Phys 2014;90(2):255–60.

15. Vilaseca I, Huerta P, Blanch JL, et al. Voice quality after CO2 laser cordectomy–what can we really expect? Head Neck 2008;30(1):43–9.

16. Tomifuji M, Araki K, Niwa K, et al. Comparison of voice quality after laser cordectomy with that after radiotherapy or chemoradiotherapy for early glottic carcinoma. ORL J Otorhinolaryngol Relat Spec 2013;75(1):18–26.

17. Remmelts AJ, Hoebers FJ, Klop WM, et al. Evaluation of lasersurgery and radiotherapy as treatment modalities in early stage laryngeal carcinoma: tumour outcome and quality of voice. Eur Arch Otorhinolaryngol 2013;270(7):2079–87.

18. Czecior E, Orecka B, Pawlas P, et al. Comparative assessment of the voice in patients treated for early glottis cancer by laser cordectomy or radiotherapy. Otolaryngol Pol 2012;66(6):407–12.

19. Cohen SM, Dupont WD, Courey MS. Quality-of-life impact of non-neoplastic voice disorders: a meta-analysis. Ann Otol Rhinol Laryngol 2006;115(2):128–34.

20. Loughran S, Calder N, MacGregor FB, et al. Quality of life and voice following endoscopic resection or radiotherapy for early glottic cancer. Clin Otolaryngol 2005;30(1):42–7.
21. Peretti G, Piazza C, Balzanelli C, et al. Preoperative and postoperative voice in Tis-T1 glottic cancer treated by endoscopic cordectomy: an additional issue for patient counseling. Ann Otol Rhinol Laryngol 2003;112(9 Pt 1):759–63.
22. Brondbo K, Benninger MS. Laser resection of T1a glottic carcinomas: results and postoperative voice quality. Acta Otolaryngol 2004;124(8):976–9.
23. Peeters AJ, van Gogh CD, Goor KM, et al. Health status and voice outcome after treatment for T1a glottic carcinoma. Eur Arch Otorhinolaryngol 2004;261(10):534–40.
24. Laoufi S, Mirghani H, Janot F, et al. Voice quality after treatment of T1a glottic cancer. Laryngoscope 2014;124(6):1398–401.
25. Roh JL, Kim DH, Kim SY, et al. Quality of life and voice in patients after laser cordectomy for Tis and T1 glottic carcinomas. Head Neck 2007;29(11):1010–6.
26. Vilaseca I, Ballesteros F, Martinez-Vidal BM, et al. Quality of life after transoral laser microresection of laryngeal cancer: a longitudinal study. J Surg Oncol 2013;108(1):52–6.
27. Carson CP, Ingrisano DR, Eggleston KD. The effect of noise on computer-aided measures of voice: a comparison of CSpeechSP and the Multi-Dimensional Voice Program software using the CSL 4300B Module and Multi-Speech for Windows. J Voice 2003;17(1):12–20.
28. Woodson GE, Cannito M. Voice analysis. In: Cummings CW, editor. Otolaryngology head and neck surgery. 3rd edition. Saint Louis (MO): Mosby-Year Book; 1998. p. 1876–90.
29. Boersma P. Should jitter be measured by peak picking or by waveform matching? Folia Phoniatr Logop 2009;61(5):305–8.
30. Luo CM, Fang TJ, Lin CY, et al. Transoral laser microsurgery elevates fundamental frequency in early glottic cancer. J Voice 2012;26(5):596–601.
31. Zeitels SM, Hillman RE, Franco RA, et al. Voice and treatment outcome from phonosurgical management of early glottic cancer. Ann Otol Rhinol Laryngol Suppl 2002;190:3–20.
32. Lundy DS, Casiano RR. "Compensatory falsetto": effects on vocal quality. J Voice 1995;9(4):439–42.
33. Stone D, McCabe P, Palme CE, et al. Voice outcomes after transoral laser microsurgery for early glottic cancer-considering signal type and smoothed cepstral peak prominence. J Voice 2015;29(3):370–81.
34. Dejonckere PH. Clinical implementation of a multidimensional basic protocol for assessing functional results of voice therapy. A preliminary study. Rev Laryngol Otol Rhinol (Bord) 2000;121(5):311–3.
35. Bielamowicz S, Kreiman J, Gerratt BR, et al. Comparison of voice analysis systems for perturbation measurement. J Speech Hear Res 1996;39(1):126–34.
36. Chu PY, Hsu YB, Lee TL, et al. Modified type III cordectomy to improve voice outcomes after transoral laser microsurgery for early glottic canser. Head Neck 2012;34(10):1422–7.
37. Ambrosch P. The role of laser microsurgery in the treatment of laryngeal cancer. Curr Opin Otolaryngol Head Neck Surg 2007;15(2):82–8.
38. Xu W, Han D, Hou L, et al. Voice function following CO2 laser microsurgery for precancerous and early-stage glottic carcinoma. Acta Otolaryngol 2007;127(6):637–41.
39. Taylor SM, Kerr P, Fung K, et al. Treatment of T1b glottic SCC: laser vs. radiation–a Canadian multicenter study. J Otolaryngol Head Neck Surg 2013;42:22.

40. Pearson BW, Salassa JR. Transoral laser microresection for cancer of the larynx involving the anterior commissure. Laryngoscope 2003;113(7):1104–12.
41. Roh JL, Kim AY. Application of mitomycin C after transoral removal of submandibular stones and sialodochoplasty. Laryngoscope 2005;115(5):915–8.
42. Roh JL, Yoon YH. Prevention of anterior glottic stenosis after transoral microresection of glottic lesions involving the anterior commissure with mitomycin C. Laryngoscope 2005;115(6):1055–9.
43. Knott PD, Milstein CF, Hicks DM, et al. Vocal outcomes after laser resection of early-stage glottic cancer with adjuvant cryotherapy. Arch Otolaryngol Head Neck Surg 2006;132(11):1226–30.
44. Cruz WP, Dedivitis RA, Rapoport A, et al. Videolaryngostroboscopy following frontolateral laryngectomy with sternohyoid flap. Ann Otol Rhinol Laryngol 2004;113(2):124–7.
45. Kerr P, Mark Taylor S, Rigby M, et al. Oncologic and voice outcomes after treatment of early glottic cancer: transoral laser microsurgery versus radiotherapy. J Otolaryngol Head Neck Surg 2012;41(6):381–8.

Voice Rehabilitation After Transoral Laser Microsurgery of the Larynx

Vyas M.N. Prasad, MSc, FRCS (ORL-HNS)[a,b,c,*], Marc Remacle, PhD, MD[a]

KEYWORDS

- Voice rehabilitation • Transoral laser microsurgery • Larynx • Voice Handicap Index

KEY POINTS

- Voice degradation is commonly seen after ELS types III to VI cordectomies.
- Anterior synechiae and glottic gap after cord resection are the commonest causes of postoperative dysphonia.
- Lichtenberger's technique is useful in treating anterior synechiae.
- Medialization thyroplasty using the Montgomery implant helps reduce the glottic gap and improve voice.

Early laryngeal cancer treatment is primarily concerned with establishing cure while preserving voice and swallow function. Treatment options include radiotherapy or surgery – open or endoscopic with similar oncologic effectiveness and identical survival rates (cause-specific survival rate ≥90%).[1] The last 20 years has demonstrated a shift in practice away from open surgical procedures to transoral surgery with satisfactory oncological outcomes.[2,3] Comparisons made between endoscopic laser microsurgery of early laryngeal cancer, open surgery and radiotherapy have also shown little difference in voice outcomes.[4,5]

Local control is similar between radiotherapy and surgery and the functional disadvantages after surgery are moderate and counterbalanced by a significantly higher rate of long-term laryngeal preservation (90.1% after radiotherapy vs 97.4% after surgery). Other advantages of the endoscopic approach include its cost-effectiveness and less limitation for future treatment options in case of failure.[6,7]

Patients undergoing less extensive microsurgery for early glottic cancer (European Laryngological Society [ELS] types I and II) are found to have mild dysphonia, which rarely requires further surgery and responds well to voice therapy. Full voice recovery

No disclosures.
[a] Department of Otolaryngology - Head and Neck Surgery, University Hospital of Louvain at Mont-Godinne, Therasse Avenue 1, Yvoir 5530, Belgium; [b] Ng Teng Fong Hospital, 1 Jurong East Street 21, Singapore; [c] Alexandra Hospital, 378 Alexandra road, Singapore
* Corresponding author.
E-mail address: vyasprasad@gmail.com

Otolaryngol Clin N Am 48 (2015) 639–653
http://dx.doi.org/10.1016/j.otc.2015.04.009
0030-6665/15/$ – see front matter © 2015 Elsevier Inc. All rights reserved.

is seen in subepithelial cordectomy (ELS type I) and is near complete in type II subligamental cordectomy. Supraglottic postoperative voice compensation is rarely if ever seen in these 2 cohorts. However, this is not the case in more extensive cordectomies, in which, although voice compensation does take place albeit at a reduced level, supraglottic contraction becomes more evident, as does compensation from part or the whole of the contralateral cord, the resulting fibrotic operated cord remnant (the neocord), or the ventricular folds.[8]

Voice degradation is seen usually after more extensive levels of cordectomy (ELS types III–V). Patients routinely undergo a minimum 6 months of voice rehabilitation with speech therapy before consideration of surgical management of dysphonia. Endoscopic and open laryngeal surgical options (thyrotomy/laryngofissure approach) are available depending on the sequelae from the primary surgical resection. We propose a step-by-step management algorithm to voice rehabilitation after endoscopic surgery (our experience) and discuss the pros and cons of the more established procedures based on experience gained in this challenging area. Open procedures and voice restoration thereafter are discussed.

Voice quality after laser microsurgery is predominantly affected by the presence of synechiae at the anterior commissure. However, the quantity of vocal cord removed and the ensuing glottic gap play significant roles in postoperative dysphonia.[2,8,9]

Several phonosurgical procedures have been developed to deal with the resulting glottic gap and anterior commissure synechiae and in so doing aim to improve phonation. We describe our experience in this regard and also take the opportunity to mention other procedures performed for these sequelae of early laryngeal surgery.

MATERIALS AND METHODS
Patients

Two hundred and fifty-one patients underwent a total of 311 CO_2 laser-assisted endoscopic cordectomies in our department between 1998 and 2012. The data of the performed procedures according to each type of cordectomy are reported in **Table 1**. Fifty-eight patients (23.1%) had more than 1 cordectomy during this period, all of whom had 2 procedures, with the exception of 1, who underwent 4. The cordectomies were classified using the revised terminology proposed in 2007 by the ELS. The revision includes a new endoscopic cordectomy (type VI) for cancers of the anterior commissure, extended to one or both of the vocal folds, without infiltration of the thyroid cartilage.[10]

All patients underwent speech therapy after establishment of the scarring process to the operated cord (ie, full development of the neocord). Total or near-total voice recovery was almost always the rule after subepithelial (type I) or subligamental (type II)

Table 1
Data according to cordectomy types

Type of Cordectomy	No. of Procedures (Total = 311) (%)	No. of Patients (Total = 251) (%)
I	138 (44.4)	64 (25.5)
II	42 (13.5)	21 (8.4)
III	42 (13.5)	32 (12.7)
IV	27 (8.7)	21 (8.4)
V	55 (17.7)	49 (19.5)
VI	7 (2.3)	6 (2.4)
Combination	—	58 (23.1)

cordectomies. Supraglottic contraction, although often observed after transmuscular (type III) cordectomy, did respond well to voice rehabilitation, assuming no anterior synechiae were present as well. More extended cordectomy rendered the ipsilateral cord nonfunctional, and voice compensation was obtained from the contralateral healthy cord or the false (ventricular) folds.[2]

Fourteen patients (5.6%) self-assessed their postoperative voice quality as insufficient, complaining of persistent dysphonia and breathiness. There were 12 men and 2 women (9 with T1 cancer and 5 with T2), with a mean age of 53.7 years (range 25–82 years) who underwent a total or extended total (13 patients) cordectomy. One patient with an anterior commissure cancer extending up to the anterior third of both cords underwent a type VI cordectomy. A type V cordectomy was performed on the 5 patients with T2 cancer as well as 3 others with T1b disease.

In addition, 10 patients developed anterior synechiae after total and extended total cordectomy or type VI cordectomy.

Voice Assessment Tools

Voice assessment was performed preoperatively and at regular intervals according to the recommendations of the Committee on Phoniatrics of the ELS.[11] We obtained complete preoperative and postoperative data on 13 of the 14 patients who underwent medialization thyroplasty and all patients who had surgery for anterior synechiae.

Self-evaluation of voice by our patients included the Voice Handicap Index (VHI) questionnaire,[12] which includes the physical, functional and emotional impact of the voice disorder and consists of 30 questions, each rated from 0 to 4, in increasing order of the severity of symptoms. Perceptual voice quality was evaluated with the GRBAS (Grade Roughness Breathiness Asthenia Strain) scale by Hirano.[13] G (overall grade) and R (roughness) (for anterior synechiae) were singled out and rated by a speech therapist with experience in voice assessment.

Aerodynamic measurements included maximum phonation time (MPT; normal range 20–25 seconds) and the phonation quotient (PQ; mL/s) (ie, the quotient obtained by dividing vital capacity with the MPT). We used the best score from 3 successive attempts of the sound "a" for the MPT at a comfortable loudness level.

Maximum fundamental frequency (Fo-high, Hz), as well as lower intensity (I-low, dB) were also calculated in medialization thyroplasty cases and the frequency range (FR, Hz) and fundamental frequency (F0) were analyzed in anterior synechiae surgery. Voice analysis was performed using the Multi Dimensional Voice Program (MDVP) (Kay Elemetrics, Lincoln Park, NJ; KayPENTAX).

Medialization Thyroplasty

Medialization thyroplasty is performed at least 6 months after cordectomy. This is considered the minimum safe period before attempted voice restoration allowing for complete healing of the larynx after laser microsurgery, formation of the neocord, assurance of no residual or recurrent disease, and voice rehabilitation accomplished with adequate voice therapy alone. The procedure is performed under general anesthesia using a laryngeal mask airway (LMA). Transnasal flexible videoendoscopy is carried out to evaluate the degree of glottic gap reduction, and this is feasible through a small valve in the joint that connects the LMA to the ventilation tube. We can assess surgical progress and completion of the thyroplasty by observing the video image captured by the camera attached to the scope without hampering the patient's ventilation.

The landmarks for creating the window in the thyroid cartilage have been slightly modified according to the different implants used over the period that the procedure has been performed. Meticulous care is taken in dissecting the inner wall of the thyroid cartilage from the fibrous neocord, ensuring close contact with the cartilage at all times, especially when the inner perichondrium was unidentifiable. Furthermore, the dissection has to be extensive enough to facilitate insertion of the implant without fibrous tissue resistance or tear. The technical difficulty of this dissection distinguishes it from medialization procedures for cord immobility, which are easier and therefore more amenable to be performed under local anesthesia (**Figs. 1** and **2**).

Three types of implants have been successfully used. The preformed Vocom hydroxyapatite implant (Smith-Nephew, Memphis, TN),[14] the Gore-Tex implant (Gore Thyroplasty Device, WL Gore and Associates, Flagstaff, AZ),[15] and the Montgomery Thyroplasty Implant System (MTIS, Boston Medical Products, Westborough, MA).[16] The Vocom implant was used primarily in 2 (14.2%) patients, the Gore-Tex in 1 (7.1%) patient, and the MTIS in 11 (78.6%) patients. A revision thyroplasty was required in only 1 case in which a Vocom implant was replaced by an MTIS.

We use quick-setting Tissucol fibrin glue (Baxter, Vienna, Austria) to cover the medialization thyroplasty window and leave a small suction drain in the wound for 24 hours before skin closure. We have found that the routine use of fibrin glue is useful in closing any potential defects between the neck and glottis. All patients are placed on postoperative broad-spectrum antibiotics (eg, co-amoxiclav) for 5 days. Voicing at a low intensity is recommended routinely after, and patients are allowed to eat the same evening of the procedure and discharged after drain removal.

Surgery for Anterior Synechiae (Lichtenberger Technique)

Our favored method to deal with anterior glottic webs is that described by Lichtenberger and Toohill.[17] The procedure is performed endoscopically under general anesthesia using suspension laryngoscopy and subglottic jet ventilation (**Fig. 3**). The laryngoscope is carefully placed at 3 to 4 mm above the anterior commissure to allow for easy placement of the silastic stent. The web is cut using a CO_2 laser with scanning facilities (Acublade system, Lumenis, Santa Clara, CA) at 10 W power in superpulse mode. The Acublade laser scanning system allows the traveling of the laser wave on a straight line. Depending on the length of the line and the type of mode selected (continuous or superpulse), the system calculates the appropriate power.[9] The cut is made in the middle of the web and care taken to extend the section up to the anterior angle of the thyroid cartilage. A cottonoid soaked with mitomycin C (2 mg/mL) is then applied twice at the surgical site for 2 minutes per application.

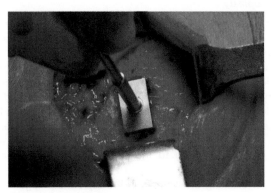

Fig. 1. Placement of window sizing gauge.

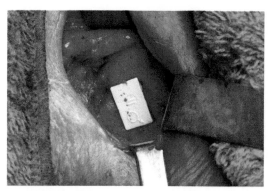

Fig. 2. Insertion of Montgomery implant.

The stent used initially was handmade and consisted of a 0.25-mm-thick silastic sheet, which was folded on itself and glued with silicone glue (Dow Corning, Midland, MI). A small tract allowing the passage of a Dermalon 2/0 thread was created by inserting a pediatric epidural needle when folding the silastic sheet. We now use a preshaped stent, the larynx anterior commissure stent (LACS, Boston Medical, Westborough, MA), which we tailor according to dimensions of the web and larynx.

Under direct endoscopic vision using a 30° rigid scope and a Lichtenberger needle holder (**Fig. 4**) (R Wolf 826750; M 954790), the LACS is fixed at the anterior commissure after sizing of the anteroposterior and superoinferior dimensions described earlier. The stent is rectangular and spans the commissure for 2 to 3 mm above and below it. The nonresorbable 00 sutures are passed through the larynx to the skin. The inferior puncture is performed first and lies below the anterior commissure and passes through the cricothyroid membrane. The superior puncture site is usually at the median of the thyroid cartilage but may vary depending on the calcification of the cartilage and may therefore be higher (eg, the base of the epiglottis) (this does not change the size of the splint). The suture is passed through a button or a silastic sheet that separates it from the skin of the neck (**Fig. 5**).

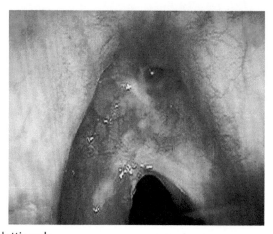

Fig. 3. Anterior glottic web.

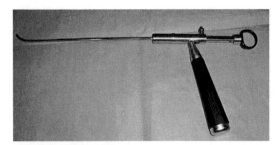

Fig. 4. Lichtenberger needle holder.

All patients are given a week's course of a broad-spectrum antibiotic (eg, co-amoxiclav), 6 weeks of twice daily proton pump inhibitors, and inhaled corticosteroids twice daily for a week. They are encouraged to rest their voice for a week postoperatively and are reviewed weekly to assess the position of the stent, which is then removed 3 weeks after the procedure (**Figs. 6** and **7**).

RESULTS

We did not observe any perioperative or immediate postoperative complications in either the medialization or the anterior web group. All patients had an unremarkable recovery, with no evidence of stridor or dyspnea. No patient required reintubation. Episodes of coughing were observed during the early recovery phase in the anterior web group, and this was successfully managed with nebulized lignocaine and antitussive medication.

Two patients required further input for delayed complications after medialization: one for a mild wound infection treated with a further course of antibiotics and the other for a minor hematoma requiring evacuation.

The average length of stay in the medialization group was 2.8 days (range 2–5 days). All patients were discharged on the same day after anterior web surgery.

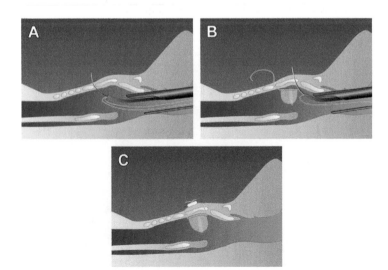

Fig. 5. (*A–C*) Stages of placement of silastic sheet.

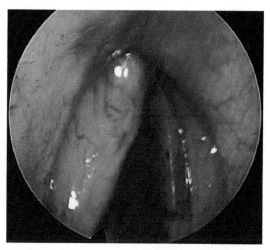

Fig. 6. View of silastic sheet after CO_2 resection of anterior glottic web.

Medialization Thyroplasty

The average interval between cordectomy and thyroplasty was 29.4 months ($\pm$ 34.2, standard deviation [SD] 8–120). Surgical placement was found to be easier with the MTIS because of its horizontal positioning and less undermining of the cephalic and caudal edge of the fibrous floor of the window (see **Figs. 1** and **2**). The Vocom hydroxyapatite implant was inserted vertically and hence was more difficult to position. The Gore-Tex implant used was a 5-mm-broad ribbon, which was inserted through the thyroid window and gradually packed into the paraglottic space until optimum medialization of the neocord was achieved. The window thereafter was covered with a small piece of silastic sheet sutured and fixed to the thyroid cartilage to avoid extrusion.

One patient experienced extrusion of the Vocom hydroxyapatite implant 10 months after surgery, having coughed it out and developing a rapidly worsening voice. A period of a month to allow for the larynx to heal adequately was instituted and an MTIS splint inserted thereafter, with resulting improvement in voice quality. No local recurrence of laryngeal cancer was seen in our series, and we noted that medialization did not modify the cord remnant and therefore does not conceal recurrence of cancer.

Laryngeal stroboscopy showed improved glottic closure during phonation, albeit irregular and incomplete, because of the fibrous edge after laser therapy. Persistent

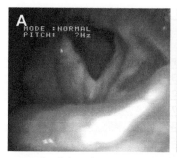
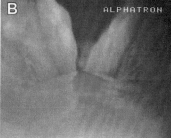

Fig. 7. Preoperative (*A*) and postoperative (*B*) views of anterior glottic web division.

vibratory asymmetry with stiffness of the fibrous neocord was also seen, with improved vibration regularity and mucosal wave of the contralateral vocal cord. Voice parameters were assessed both subjectively and objectively and comparison made before and after surgery. A reduction was seen in the following parameters: (1) VHI from 50.5 to 39.4; (2) G, 2.4 to 2; (3) maximum fundamental frequency (Fo-high) from 338.7 to 242.4 Hz; (4) lower intensity (I-low) 60 to 58 dB; and (5) PQ from 1144.9 to 544.9 mL/s (**Table 2**). MPT was increased from 6.2 to 7.3 seconds. There was a statistically significant difference for the VHI scores and G grading. The difference in PQ was not statistically significant but was, however, diminished by more than half the preoperative value. Objective acoustical analysis showed a decrease in Fo at a comfortable speaking voice. Subjectively, all patients presented with less vocal fatigue and required less effort in supporting phonation over the course of the day.

A further subgroup analysis of voice assessment parameters and type of cordectomy showed greater decrease in VHI in patients who underwent type IV cordectomy. Overall, grade G changed equally in type IV and V cordectomy but neither VHI nor G changed in the type VI category (**Table 3**).

Anterior Synechial Surgery

None of the patients treated had or needed to have a tracheostomy at any point and all tolerated the stent well. Removal of the stent was performed at 3 weeks under general anesthesia; follow-up visits took place at 1 and 3 months after surgery and thereafter at variable intervals, depending on the underlying disease. The mean follow-up was 48.4 months (3–87 months). Postoperative laryngoscopy showed no residual web in any of the patients.

Speech therapy was initiated after removal of the stent in all patients. Statistical voice analysis of the voice parameters comparing the results at the last follow-up with those recorded before surgery (**Table 4**) showed a statistically significant improvement in the overall grade G (G preoperatively, 2; postoperatively; 1; $P = .035$).

DISCUSSION

Early glottic cancers (ie, T1 and T2) have been shown to be effectively cured by total or extended cordectomies. However, these procedures have been shown to result in glottic defects and anterior synechiae, which affect voice quality. Speech therapy alone is not effective in restoring a normal voice in such cases, and hence, in carefully selected and motivated patients, laryngeal framework or anterior web surgery is recommended.

Table 2
Voice assessment (mean ± SD) in 13 patients

Variables	Preoperative Values (Mean ± SD)	Postoperative Values (Mean ± SD)	P Values
VHI	50.5 ± 23.7	39.4 ± 27	.049
G	2.4 ± 0.7	2 ± 0.6	.018
MPT	6.2 ± 2.5	7.3 ± 2.8	.193
Fo-high	338.7 ± 101.1	242.4 ± 141.3	.869
I-low	60 ± 11.2	58 ± 13	.365
PQ	1144.9 ± 1307.2	544.9 ± 287.8	.149

Table 3
Statistically significant changes of voice assessment parameters according to cordectomy type

Cordectomy Type	DVHI, Mean (SD)	DG, Mean (SD)
IV	15.2 (28.5)	0.4 (0.5)
V	6.4 (8.9)	0.4 (0.5)
VI	0	0

Six-Month Interval

We usually wait 6 months before consideration of laryngeal framework intervention. This allows the patient to have rested the larynx, forming a stable scarred neocord and thereafter undergoing speech therapy. This strategy also leaves a sufficient interval to assess for recurrence. Surgery is advocated only when posttherapy voice outcomes do not meet the desired voice requirements but is nevertheless not always instituted because of patient preference.

Injection

Our findings suggest that laryngeal framework surgery is more effective than intracordal injections.[18] Our attempts to close the glottic gap using collagen injections failed because the vocal structure was no longer present and therefore the injectable material could no longer be enclosed within the Reinke space. Other injectables such as silicone, fat, and bioplastic, despite being successful in vocal cord immobility surgery, were found unsuitable, because they are injected between the cartilage and the vocal cord, which in the case of the total or extended cordectomy is not possible.[19,20] Therefore, injection laryngoplasty[18] after total or extended cordectomy was found to be futile given the tight scar tissue replacing the ligamentous cord and muscle. However, we do use hyaluronic acid in cases in which scarring is minimal (ie, surgical removal of small lesions; benign or malignant/iatrogenic injury).

Voice Assessment

Subjective and objective voice measures were used to assess voice outcome. We found that the VHI questionnaire better reflected patients' perception of voice outcome as did the rater-based GRBAS severity grade compared with objective parameters from acoustical analysis. There is no doubt that the VHI is a well-organized, qualified instrument that provides more perception into voice-related issues in daily life of patients treated for early glottic cancer than a single report of voice quality. It can therefore provide useful data to explain why patients with similar dysphonia characteristics can have different handicap severity indices.

Table 4
Voice parameters preoperatively and postoperatively

Variables	Preoperative Values	Postoperative Values	P
G	2	1	.035
R	2	1	.083
VHI	54	46	.263
MPT (s)	11.31	11.28	1
PQ (mL/s)	327	395	.722
FR (Hz)	145	185	.286
F0 (Hz)	211	222	.944

Objective evaluation in our medialization thyroplasty cohort showed a reduced Fo, possibly correlating with a reduction of supraglottic contraction anteroposteriorly or laterally from the ventricular folds. Although not strictly significant, we did see a trend of improvement in the aerodynamic parameters, MPT and PQ, which we hope in a future larger series will reach statistical significance. As for our anterior synechiae group, objective voice parameters were not significantly improved, because of the limited numbers and the persistence of scarred vocal folds, despite resection of the web and improvement in respiration.

Bertino and colleagues[21] showed no difference in voice quality after cordectomy with or without reconstruction using acoustic analysis. However, Zeitels and colleagues[22] reported positive results after glottic reconstruction after cordectomy based on digitized acoustic measurements. This discrepancy is dependent on the unstable neocord vibration after endoscopic cordectomy and this may render variability to some digitized voice analyses.

Scales for perceptual evaluation[9,23] and basic aerodynamic measurements (MPT, PQ) remain valuable.[24] Studies that included these tools[9,24,25] showed improvement after reconstruction. Sittel and colleagues[25] used a dysphonia index that ranged from 0 (normal) to 3 (aphonia), which included objective parameters as well as expert voice ratings and patient's perception.

Open Surgery: Flaps and Laryngofissure

Open surgery for early glottic cancer using a thyrotomy (laryngofissure) approach[21,26–32] to both resect the tumor and also reconstruct the defect has been well described using the sternohyoid muscle[33,34] or the ventricular band (false cord vocal flap) with or without fat or cartilage interposition. Bipedicled strap muscle transposition flaps,[35] bilateral omohyoid muscle flaps,[30] vestibular fold flaps[21,31] and composite myomucosal reconstruction[32] have been described but require major dissection without significantly better voice results.

Medialization Thyroplasty

Isshiki first described the thyroplasty type I in 1974,[18] and this procedure is now classified as medialization thyroplasty by the Phonosurgery Committee of the ELS.[36] A variety of indications have emerged for this popular procedure, including the treatment of unilateral vocal fold palsy, congenital vocal atrophy, sulcus, and scarring,[37] and many techniques have been proposed for the improvement of glottic incompetence after CO_2 laser transoral cordectomy, with varying advantages and disadvantages.

Over the years, we have used many different types of prosthetic materials, such as thyroid cartilage, titanium, hydroxyapatite, silicone, and Gore-Tex.[24,38] Thyroid cartilage was found to be cumbersome, because of its vertical position perpendicular to the plane of the vocal neocord and its resorption with time. Vocom hydroxyapatite was found to be more difficult to handle and also had a vertical configuration when inserted.[14] The Friedrich titanium implant can be too rigid in cordectomy cases.[39] The Montgomery (MTIS) implant has the advantage of being flexible, easy to handle, and with rounded edges, which do not traumatize the fibrous neocord. Gore-Tex has been advocated by several investigators because of its ease of handling, placement in complex defects, flexibility, and in vivo adjustability.[15]

SYNECHIAE OF THE ANTERIOR LARYNX

The development of anterior glottic webs (synechiae) postcordectomy (ELS type Va, VI) is another sequela of endolaryngeal laser surgery for early cancers of the glottis and presents with several challenges, which include management of dysphonia and dyspnea. Several treatment modalities have been reported in the literature, both open and closed.[40] However, none achieves perfect morphologic or functional results. Mucosal and skin flaps have also been described to cover the involved surface of the vocal folds.[41-44] We favor the transoral inside-out approach as described by Lichtenberger using a silastic stent, LACS, which has been also described as a keel.[45] Previous descriptions also include an outside-in technique, which we find more cumbersome.[17,46-48]

Our management of these webs is dependent on the thickness and length and the impact they have on voice and breathing. In general, most postoperative iatrogenically caused webs in the context of laser microsurgery are well formed, relatively thick, and extend up to the anterior third of the vocal cord. Our experience in this adult population has been relatively successful with the use of the endoscopic CO_2 laser section of the web, application of mitomycin C, and placement of a silastic splint in the anterior commissure for 3 weeks, as described by Lichtenberger.

Our results have been positive in improving the morphology of the anterior glottis and rater-related overall grade G (according to the Hirano scale) but with little improvement in the voice of the patient on the VHI.

Mitomycin C

Mitomycin C is an antimitotic agent, which has been used for more than 20 years in ophthalmology for the topical treatment of pterygium and scars arising after glaucoma surgery.[49,50] Several studies have reported encouraging results in the treatment of upper aerodigestive tract webs and stenosis.[51-56] It has also been used successfully in the prevention of restenosis in sinus meatotomies[52] and choanal atresia.[53] In selected cases, it has obviated stent/keel placement.[57]

Although there are varying concentrations and durations of application in the literature,[51-56] we have had good results using a concentration of 2 mg/mL (as described by P. Monnier, personal communication, 1999) for 2 minutes without washing the chemical away. This step was repeated once more in our series (ie, performed twice in total).

Speech Therapy

We routinely advocate speech therapy before making a decision on embarking on surgery and postoperatively. Sittel and colleagues[9] suggest no evidence of significant benefit from speech therapy after cordectomy, but we believe that it does help in preventing ineffective supraglottic hyperkinetic dysfunction, seen more commonly in type I and II cordectomies. Furthermore, speech therapy has been shown to strengthen glottic closure and loudness of voice, improve efficiency of breath expenditure, increase articulation skill and intelligibility of speech, recognize and compensate for hearing loss, and aid patients in the reduction of detrimental environmental influences and adjusting to their environmental requirements.[58]

Anesthetic Considerations

Laryngeal framework surgery to medialize the cord can be performed using several techniques and under either local or general anesthesia. We advocate the use of general anesthesia in the case of glottic gap correction after cordectomy, because the procedure is longer and requires more dissection as opposed to medialization as a result of cord immobility. The use of the LMA and fiber-optic videolaryngoscopy through it allows for excellent control of medialization without compromising ventilation.

We used an automated jet ventilation delivery system passed subglottically for surgery on anterior synechiae. This system allowed for adequate access to the larynx and instrumentation using the Lichtenberger needle holder and 30° rigid endoscope.

SUMMARY

Voice rehabilitation after transoral laser microsurgery to the larynx is challenging. We wait at least 6 months before embarking on any surgical intervention. Only a few patients (14 patients, 5.6%) after total or extended cordectomy requested voice restoration. We found that subjective perception of voice using VHI in medialization thyroplasty was significantly better. In this regard, self-evaluation questionnaires such as the VHI are probably more useful tools along with stroboscopy for voice assessment.

Medialization thyroplasty with careful elevation of the fibrous tissue from the inner surface of the thyroid cartilage is critical in achieving success. We preferred the MTIS implant in most cases, although the Gore-Tex implant is useful in more scarred complex defects. Transoral LACS placement (Lichtenberger technique) after laser-assisted sectioning of anterior synechiae with application of mitomycin C is an effective procedure for anterior synechiae.

REFERENCES

1. Bron LP, Soldati D, Zouhair A, et al. Treatment of early stage squamous-cell carcinoma of the glottic larynx: endoscopic surgery or cricohyoidoepiglottopexy versus radiotherapy. Head Neck 2001;23(10):823–9.
2. Remacle M, Lawson G, Jamart J, et al. CO_2 laser in the diagnosis and treatment of early cancer of the vocal fold. Eur Arch Otorhinolaryngol 1997;254:169–76.
3. Silver CE, Beitler JJ, Shaha AR, et al. Current trends in initial management of laryngeal cancer: the declining use of open surgery. Eur Arch Otorhinolaryngol 2009;266:1333–52.
4. Morris MR, Canonico D, Blank C. A critical review of radiotherapy in the management of T1 glottic carcinoma. Am J Otolaryngol 1994;15(4):276–80.
5. Delsupehe KG, Zink I, Lejaegere M, et al. Voice quality after narrow-margin laser cordectomy compared with laryngeal irradiation. Otolaryngol Head and Neck Surg 1999;121:528–33.
6. Peretti G, Nicolai P, De Zinis LOR, et al. Endoscopic CO_2 laser excision for Tis, T1 and T2 glottic carcinomas: cure rates and prognostic factors. Otolaryngol Head and Neck Surg 2000;123:124–31.
7. Goor KM, Peeters AJGE, Mahieu HF, et al. Cordectomy by CO_2 laser or radiotherapy for small T1a glottic carcinomas: costs, local control, survival, quality of life and voice quality. Head Neck 2007;2:128–36.
8. Peretti G, Piazza C, Balzanelli C, et al. Preoperative and postoperative voice in Tis-T1 glottic cancer treated by endoscopic cordectomy: an additional issue for patient counselling. Ann Otol Rhinol Laryngol 2003;112:759–63.
9. Sittel C, Eckel HE, Eschenburg C. Phonatory results after laser surgery for glottic carcinoma. Otolaryngol Head Neck Surg 1998;119:418–24.
10. Remacle M, Van Haverbeke C, Eckel H, et al. Proposal for revision of the European Laryngological Society classification of endoscopic cordectomies. Eur Arch Otorhinolaryngol 2007;264:499–504.
11. DeJonckere PH, Bradley P, Clemente P, et al. A basic protocol for functional voice pathology, especially for measuring the efficacy of (phonosurgical) treatments and evaluating new assessment techniques. Guidelines elaborated by the

Committee on Phoniatrics of the European Laryngological Society (ELS). Eur Arch Otorhinolaryngol 2001;258:77–82.

12. Jacobson BH, Johnson A, Grywalsky C, et al. The voice handicap index (VHI): development and validation. Am J Speech Lang Pathol 1997;6:66–70.

13. Hirano M. Clinical examination of voice. New York: Springer; 1981.

14. Cummings CW, Purcell LL, Flint PW. Hydroxylapatite laryngeal implants for medialization. Preliminary report. Ann Otol Rhinol Laryngol 1993;102:843–51.

15. Zeitels SM, Mauri M, Dailey SH. Medialization laryngoplasty with Gore-Tex for voice restoration secondary to glottal incompetence: indications and observations. Ann Otol Rhinol Laryngol 2003;112(2):180–4.

16. Montgomery WW, Montgomery SK. Montgomery thyroplasty implant system. Ann Otol Rhinol Laryngol Suppl 1997;170:1–16.

17. Lichtenberger G, Toohill RJ. New keel fixing technique for endoscopic repair of anterior commissure webs. Laryngoscope 1994;104(6 Pt 1):771–4.

18. Ford CN, Bless DM. Selected problems treated by vocal fold injection of collagen. Am J Otolaryngol 1993;14:257–61.

19. Remacle M, Marbaix E. Further morphological studies on collagen injected into canine vocal folds. Ann Otol Rhinol Laryngol 1991;100:1007–14.

20. Remacle M, Lawson G, Keghian J, et al. Use of injectable autologous collagen for correcting glottic gaps: initial results. J Voice 1999;13:280–8.

21. Bertino G, Bellomo A, Ferrero FE, et al. Acoustic analysis of voice quality with or without false vocal cord displacement after cordectomy. J Voice 2001;15(1):131–40.

22. Zeitels SM, Hillman RE, Franco RA, et al. Voice and treatment outcome from phonosurgical management of early glottic cancer. Ann Otol Rhinol Laryngol Suppl 2002;190:3–20.

23. Yamaguchi H, Shrivastav R, Andrews ML, et al. A comparison of voice quality ratings made by Japanese and American listeners using the GRBAS scale. Folia Phoniatr Logop 2003;55(3):147–57.

24. Remacle M, Lawson G, Hedayat A, et al. Medialization framework surgery for voice improvement after endoscopic cordectomy. Eur Arch Otorhinolaryngol 2001;258:267–71.

25. Sittel C, Friedrich G, Zorowka P, et al. Surgical voice rehabilitation after laser surgery for glottic carcinoma. Ann Otol Rhinol Laryngol 2002;111(6):493–9.

26. Neel HB, Devine KD, DeSanto LW. Laryngofissure and cordectomy for early cordal carcinoma: outcome in 182 patients. Otolaryngol Head and Neck Surg 1980; 88:79–84.

27. Daly JF, Kwok FM. Laryngofissure and cordectomy. Laryngoscope 1975;85: 1290–7.

28. Friedman M, Toriuni DM. Glottic reconstruction following hemilaryngectomy: false cord advancement flap. Laryngoscope 1987;97:882–4.

29. Tucker HM, Wood BG, Levine H, et al. Glottic reconstruction after near total laryngectomy. Laryngoscope 1979;89:609–18.

30. Calcaterra TC. Bilateral omohyoid muscle flap reconstruction for anterior commissure cancer. Laryngoscope 1987;97(7 Pt 1):810–3.

31. Martins Mamede RC, Ricz HM, Guiar-Ricz LN, et al. Vestibular fold flap for postcordectomy laryngeal reconstruction. Otolaryngol Head Neck Surg 2005;132(3): 478–83.

32. Milutinoivc Z. Composite myo-mucosal reconstruction of the vocal fold. Eur Arch Otolaryngol 1995;252(2):119–22.

33. Hirano M. A technique for glottic reconstruction following vertical partial laryngectomy. Auris Nasus Larynx 1978;5:63–70.

34. Pech A, Thomassin JM, Goubert JL, et al. Glottic reconstruction with a flap of thyroid perichondrium. Ann Otolaryngol Chir Cervicofac 1984;101:319–22 [in French].
35. Su CY, Chuang HC, Tsai SS, et al. Bipedicled strap muscle transposition for vocal fold deficit after laser cordectomy in early glottic cancer patients. Laryngoscope 2005;115(3):528–33.
36. Friedrich G, de Jong F, Mahieu HF, et al. Laryngeal framework surgery: a proposal for classification and nomenclature by the Phonosurgery Committee of the European Laryngological Society. Eur Arch Otolaryngol 2001;258:389–96.
37. Zeitels SM, Jarboe J, Franco RA. Phonosurgical reconstruction of early glottic cancer. Laryngoscope 2001;111:1862–5.
38. Remacle M, Lawson G, Morsomme D, et al. Reconstruction of glottic defects after endoscopic cordectomy: voice outcome. Otolaryngol Clin North Am 2006;39:191–204.
39. Friedrich G. Titanium vocal fold implant: introducing a novel implant system for external vocal fold medialization. Ann Otol Rhinol Laryngol 1999;113:853–8.
40. Montgomery WW, Montgomery SK. Manual for use of Montgomery laryngeal, tracheal, and esophageal prostheses: update 1990. Ann Otol Rhinol Laryngol Suppl 1990;150:2–28.
41. Isshiki N, Taira T, Nose K, et al. Surgical treatment of laryngeal web with mucosa graft. Ann Otol Rhinol Laryngol 1991;100:95–100.
42. Schweinfurth J. Single-stage, stentless endoscopic repair of the anterior glottic webs. Laryngoscope 2002;112:933–5.
43. Wang Z, Pankratov MM, Rebeiz EE, et al. Endoscopic diode laser welding of mucosal grafts on the larynx: a new technique. Laryngoscope 1995;105:49–52.
44. Rosen CA, Simpson CB. Anterior glottis web. Chapter 26. In: Operative techniques in laryngology. Berlin: Springer; 2008. p. 159–64.
45. Parker DA, Das Gupta AR. An endoscopic silastic keel for anterior glottis webs. J Laryngol Otol 1987;101:1055–61.
46. Casiano RR, Lundy DS. Outpatient transoral laser vaporization of anterior glottic webs and keel placement: risks of airway compromise. J Voice 1998;12(4):536–9.
47. Dedo HH. Endoscopic Teflon keel for anterior glottic web. Ann Otol Rhinol Laryngol 1979;88(4 Pt 1):467–73.
48. Tucker HM. Laryngeal webs–management of specific lesions. Surgery for phonatory disorders. New York: Churchill Livingstone; 1981.
49. Singh G, Wilson MR, Foster CS. Mitomycin eye drops as a treatment of pterygium. Ophthalmology 1988;95:813–21.
50. Chen CW, Huang HT, Blair JS, et al. Trabeculectomy with simultaneous topical application of mitomycin C in refractory glaucoma. J Ocul Pharmacol 1990;6:175–82.
51. De Mones E, Lagarde F, Hans S, et al. Mitomycin C: prevention and treatment of anterior glottic synechiae. Ann Otolaryngol Chir Cervicofac 2004;121:229–34.
52. Chung JH, Cosenza MJ, Rahbar R, et al. Mitomycin C for the prevention of adhesion formation after endoscopic sinus surgery: a randomized, controlled study. Otolaryngol Head Neck Surg 2002;126:468–74.
53. Holland BW, McGuirt WF. Surgical management of choanal atresia: improvement outcome using mitomycin. Arch Otolaryngol Head Neck Surg 2001;127:1375–80.
54. Hartnick CJ, Hartley BE, Lacy PD, et al. Topical mitomycin application after laryngotracheal reconstruction. Arch Otolaryngol Head Neck Surg 2001;127:1260–4.

55. Rahbar R, Jones DT, Roberson DW, et al. The role of mitomycin in the prevention and treatment of scar formation in the pediatric aerodigestive tract. Arch Otolaryngol Head Neck Surg 2002;128:401–6.

56. Rahbar R, Shapshay SM, Healy GB. Mitomycin: effects on laryngeal and tracheal stenosis, benefits and complications. Ann Otol Rhinol Laryngol 2001;10:1–6.

57. Unal M. The successful management of congenital laryngeal web with endoscopic lysis and topical mitomycin-C. Int J Pediatr Otorhinolaryngol 2004;68(2): 231–5.

58. Moore GP. Voice problems following limited surgical excision. Laryngoscope 1975;85(4):619–25.

Preserving and Restoring Function in Advanced Laryngeal Cancer

Quality of Life After Conservation Surgery for Laryngeal Cancer

Babak Sadoughi, MD*

KEYWORDS

- Laryngeal cancer • Quality of life • Total laryngectomy • Partial laryngectomy
- Conservation laryngeal surgery • Organ preservation

KEY POINTS

- Any treatment modality of laryngeal carcinoma can have effects on laryngeal function, and the impact of treatment on function has to be carefully weighed against its oncologic benefit.
- Quality of life (QOL) after treatment should be viewed as an independent outcome variable to be included in the management algorithm.
- Total laryngectomy (TL) is a radical procedure with significant QOL-related morbidity, and exploring alternative management possibilities has been the basis for the development of organ preservation strategies.
- Conservation laryngeal surgery has wide applications in the management of laryngeal cancer.
- Transoral laser microsurgery (TLM) and transcervical partial laryngectomy procedures offer significant QOL advantages when compared with total laryngectomy and should be considered as feasible treatment options in appropriately selected cases of early, advanced, and recurrent laryngeal cancer.

OVERVIEW

Laryngeal cancer has a singular position as a life-threatening condition affecting a complex organ of utmost functional importance. The critical role of the larynx in the maintenance of such cardinal physiologic functions as phonation, regulation of respiratory airflow, and airway protection during deglutition invariably prompts crucial dilemmas when a malignant neoplasm affects this organ. Although TL is still viewed as the ablative procedure of reference, it remains a radical procedure with significant

Disclosures/Conflicts of Interest: None.
* Department of Otolaryngology-Head and Neck Surgery, The Sean Parker Institute for the Voice, Weill Cornell Medical College, 1305 York Avenue, 5th Floor, New York, NY 10021, USA.
E-mail address: bas9049@med.cornell.edu

Otolaryngol Clin N Am 48 (2015) 655–665
http://dx.doi.org/10.1016/j.otc.2015.04.010
0030-6665/15/$ – see front matter © 2015 Elsevier Inc. All rights reserved.

consequences on various qualitative measures of human performance and considerable rehabilitation requirements.

Nonsurgical treatment modalities gained importance in the era of organ preservation protocols but demonstrated their own shortcomings with long-term morbidity issues and added difficulty in the management of treatment failure. After timid beginnings fraught by harsh criticism, transoral microlaryngeal surgery rapidly gained popularity as an oncologically valid alternative to radiation therapy for early glottic lesions, relegating time-honored open partial laryngectomy approaches to a status of quasi-irrelevance given their higher morbidity. The latter are now undergoing a genuine revival as alternative means to either address advanced-stage disease or propose salvage management after radiation failure.

After placing the emphasis of management strategies on oncologic outcomes, and subsequently, on raw functional outcomes, QOL assessments have only recently become a focus of attention. QOL does not necessarily correlate with adequacy of objective functional parameters or with the elementary indicators of oncologic control, but in fact embodies a less-tangible amalgamation of both objective and subjective factors. The increasing complexity of the decision-making process in the management of laryngeal cancer only underscores the importance of an individualized approach, tailored to the patient's lesion, expectations, and overall health status.

Importance of Quality of Life in the Management Algorithm

The treatment of any malignancy relies primarily on an oncologically validated model of disease control, with a particular emphasis on local control or regional control while focusing on prolonged survival as the ultimate goal. This paradigm was historically the basis to justify the most radical therapeutic approaches, often sacrificing some or all function—and frequently QOL—to increased survival. In addition, a once paternalistic perspective of the practice of medicine served to contribute to substituting patient autonomy with expert clinical judgment.

In more recent times, QOL as reported by the patient, regardless of correlation with clinical or objective parameters of health, is viewed as a factor of paramount importance. In a survey of otolaryngologists, Demez and Moreau[1] noted that most practitioners considered QOL, particularly relating to pain and breathing, to be at least as important as survival in the management of head and neck cancers, and that the physician's perception of patient QOL had an influence on the proposed choice of treatment. In another survey of healthy professionals faced with a hypothetical personal diagnosis of advanced laryngeal cancer, 20% of respondents declared they would opt for a treatment modality that would provide them with a preserved voice quality over one that would provide improved survival at the detriment of voice function.[2] These sporadic results may admittedly not be extrapolated into algorithms but reflect the importance of tailoring treatment strategies to each patient's particular situation.

RELEVANT PROBLEMS
Impact of Total Laryngectomy on Quality of Life

The decision to undergo a TL implies the creation of an irreversible diversion of the tracheal airway to a permanent cervical stoma, resulting in the inability to use the remaining upper airway structures (oral, nasal, and pharyngeal cavities) for respiratory exchanges. As a consequence, the laryngectomee also becomes dependent on routine stomal care measures and devices to prevent excessive bronchorrhea, airway obstruction, and pulmonary complications. An often-overlooked complaint that ensues is the loss of olfactory faculties.[3] Although this deficit can be addressed through simple rehabilitation measures, caregivers commonly dismiss it as a minor and inevitable outcome of TL.[4]

The negative effects of TL on QOL are difficult to mitigate. Despite the eventual adjustment of patients to their new status, a TL is commonly experienced as a form of physical mutilation associated with severe psychosocial effects that do not seem to improve over time.[5–8] The adjunction of radiation therapy seems to amplify the detrimental effects of TL on QOL.[3]

The mere need for a permanent stoma plays a significant role in the deterioration of perceptual QOL measures, presumably because of the heavy social stigma and psychological adaptation needs associated with it.[9] Potter and Birchall[10] queried a population of laryngectomees on their interest in a possible restoration of function by laryngeal transplant and found that 75% of respondents would be agreeable to a transplant under ideal circumstances. However, the proportion of potential volunteers dropped to 58.9% if a stoma was to be retained after transplant, illustrating the significant contribution of the stoma to the perceived morbidity of TL.[10]

Morbidity of Radiation Therapy

The classic alternative to radical surgical management of laryngeal cancer is external beam radiation therapy, with the option of concurrent radiosensitizing systemic chemotherapy. A seminal 1991 Veterans Affairs study brought the concept of organ preservation into the spotlight, by proposing an ingenuous selection protocol of candidates for curative nonsurgical treatment modalities.[11] Two decades later, the vast adoption of nonsurgical treatment of laryngeal cancer has revealed significant shortcomings with respect to the suboptimal residual function of an otherwise anatomically intact organ, and the difficulty in addressing persistent or recurrent disease with non radical surgical treatment once radiation is delivered. Thus, the term 'organ preservation' bears only relative value and should be interpreted with caution, because the functional status of an organ is just as important as its mere presence.[12]

When used as an adjuvant modality after surgical management, radiation therapy has independent supplemental impact on QOL: Vilaseca and colleagues[13] noted a negative influence of radiation therapy and neck dissection on disease-specific QOL after TLM for early to intermediate laryngeal carcinoma; similarly, the QOL relating to voice and swallowing functions after TL was noted to be negatively affected by radiotherapy.[3,14]

THE TRANSORAL ALTERNATIVE
Transoral Laser Microsurgery

TLM rapidly emerged as an alternative, minimally invasive surgical modality offering excellent oncologic outcomes and ease of recovery.[15] Aside from cases in which anatomic or technical limitations render TLM unfeasible, the main reservation associated with the technique lies in deterioration of voice function, directly linked to the extent of glottic tissue resected. Nevertheless, despite variable outcomes with respect to voice quality, TLM seems to retain notable advantages in QOL outcomes. When compared with radiotherapy, Luo and colleagues[16] found that although TLM resulted in an increase in the fundamental frequency of the voice, the voice-related QOL was similar and patients undergoing TLM enjoyed better overall communication abilities; Oridate and colleagues[17] had previously observed similar reported voice-related QOL measures, with significantly worse scores after TL compared with TLM or radiotherapy.

One specific drawback of TLM is a prolonged postoperative interval of recovery of voice stability, estimated to range from 3 to 6 months. Therefore any assessment or comparison of definitive functional outcomes after TLM should not take place before this recovery period has elapsed.[18]

Early Glottic Carcinoma

Early malignancy of the glottis certainly exemplifies a domain in which the purported QOL benefits of minimally invasive surgery have their most remarkable illustration. Oncologic outcomes and voice-related QOL were found to be comparable between TLM and external beam therapy in stage I and II glottic carcinoma.[19,20] Similarly, a systematic review performed by Spielmann and colleagues[21] concluded that the voice quality and QOL were comparable between TLM and radiotherapy, although the statistical power of the review was noted to be fairly low. Another systematic review by van Loon and colleagues[22] also recognized the difficulty to attain sufficient statistical power in comparing the modalities and acknowledged the need to standardize methodology to improve the reliability of comparative studies.

The minimally invasive characteristic of TLM is of particular interest when the patient's general state of health or comorbidities prompt concerns as to their amenability to radiation therapy or radical surgery. For instance, excellent oncologic outcomes and ease of recovery have been noted to make TLM a beneficial alternative to radiation therapy in the elderly.[23] Furthermore, although there have been anecdotal reports of robot-assisted transoral partial laryngectomy, those were limited to supraglottic resections due to the spatial constraints associated with the cumbersome robotic systems currently available. It is reasonable to anticipate that robotic surgery will hold greater promises for laryngeal surgery as increasingly miniaturized systems are developed in the future.

Finally, cost considerations may also weigh in the choice of modality. In a Canadian retrospective study, the treatment of early glottic carcinoma with definitive external beam radiation therapy was found to be 4 times as costly as single-modality management with TLM.[24] Although that absolute ratio may not be exactly representative of every health care system worldwide, it is safe to presume that, universally, the requisite resources, equipment, time, and personnel commitments of a complete modern radiation treatment regimen represent significantly greater expenditures than what is needed to perform a single TLM procedure followed by a brief hospital admission. However the in-depth economic analysis that is required to corroborate this hypothesis is beyond the scope of this article.

CLINICAL OUTCOMES OF OPEN PARTIAL LARYNGECTOMY
Oncologic Outcomes

The rapid expansion of nonsurgical organ preservation protocols in the 1990s induced a decrease in the use of open partial laryngectomy in the management of laryngeal carcinoma. The broad adoption of the TLM approach generated further momentum for the decline of transcervical partial resection in the early 2000s.[25]

While one might have anticipated a gradual disappearance of open partial laryngectomy, the technique has instead been enjoying an actual resurgence in the past few years, albeit limited to select specialized centers. On one hand, this trend can be explained by growing numbers of postradiation treatment failures and the often suboptimal efficacy of nonsurgical treatment regimens bearing severe toxicity. Some even expressed concern about presumably decreasing survival rates with nonsurgical treatment being illustrative of missed opportunities for conservation surgery approaches,[26] facing strong rebuttals from advocates of nonsurgical treatment.[27,28]

On the other hand, higher patient and provider expectations with respect to QOL outcomes have also driven a reevaluation of TL alternatives, whether in the management of advanced laryngeal carcinoma or for salvage ablation of recurrent carcinoma. The latter situation has become the preferred indication of open partial laryngectomy, which is no longer justified in the setting of its original applications. A typical example would be a T1 or T2 lesion of the anterior glottic commissure, which would nowadays be better addressed transorally than by supracricoid partial laryngectomy (SCPL) as it used to be.[29] The use of SCPL for T3 and T4 laryngeal lesions has been noted to produce adequate oncologic outcomes,[30] and open partial laryngectomy has been deemed equivalent to radiation therapy with respect to overall survival, voice quality, and stoma avoidance rate when used to manage T3N0 lesions of the glottis.[31] Lastly, a retrospective analysis of TL surgical specimens by Weinstein and colleagues[32] demonstrated that a nonnegligible subset of the examined tumors would have been possible candidates for SCPL and thus, organ conservation treatment, implying that TL is probably an overused procedure.

Another phenomenon suspected to be an effect of the development of nonsurgical modalities for laryngeal cancer has been a notable decline in survival rates. In a multicenter study by Bussu and colleagues,[33] SCPL with cricohyoidopexy was able to produce survival rates similar to concurrent chemoradiation and greater rates of laryngeal preservation, albeit with the recognition that the procedure was only feasible in selected cases and that concurrent chemoradiation still enjoyed vast applicability. Qian and colleagues[34] noted that the judicious use of adjuvant therapy after partial laryngectomy afforded greater survival than nonsurgical multimodality treatment of advanced tumors.

Quality of Life Outcomes

After decades of controversy, open partial laryngectomy eventually gained definitive acceptance as a safe oncologic alternative to TL in the right indications. However, several factors have precluded widespread adoption of partial laryngectomy as a routine tool in the armamentarium of the head and neck surgical oncologist.

First, when posing a surgical indication, the obligation to follow strict patient selection criteria naturally makes partial laryngectomy the exception rather than the rule; remarkably, although the setting of open partial laryngectomy may be shifting from a primary ablative approach to an alternative or salvage approach, the principal selection criteria remain largely unchanged in either context with respect to amenable tumor boundaries, as well as anatomic and functional contraindications; notably, preserving the cricoid cartilage and at least 1 functional cricoarytenoid unit is of paramount importance (**Box 1**). In addition, transcervical partial laryngectomy procedures entail significant technical challenges at all levels: initial patient and lesion evaluation, discussion of risks and alternatives, skillful execution of the procedure, and postoperative management needs present daunting pitfalls and complexity to the head and neck surgeon lacking relevant experience. This aspect is amplified by an ongoing attrition of surgeons well versed in conservation surgery of the larynx, which, in turn, results in the virtual absence of these techniques in modern otolaryngology–head and neck surgery training curricula, thereby turning transcervical partial laryngectomy into a lost art. However, such issues are alleviated by the fact that laryngeal cancer is a steadily declining disease entity and its management would probably be adequately served by a limited number of highly specialized centers.

Notwithstanding the above-listed factors, the foremost impediment to broader use of transcervical conservation laryngeal surgery probably lies in the excessive variability in the perception and accounts of the postoperative QOL associated with it.

Box 1
Conventional contraindications of organ-sparing surgery of the larynx

- Subglottic extension greater than 10 mm anteriorly, greater than 5 mm laterally, and greater than 2 mm posteriorly
- Arytenoid fixation
- Massive preepiglottic space invasion with vallecular projection
- Deep extension into pharyngeal wall, vallecula, and base of tongue
- Involvement of postcricoid or interarytenoid region
- Invasion of cricoid cartilage
- Extralaryngeal extension
- Poor cardiorespiratory reserve or performance status

Multiple descriptive studies have supported the acceptable QOL resulting from SCPL.[35,36] Others recognize the alteration of voice quality that ensues after partial laryngectomy but still advocate for open conservation techniques given the maintenance of near-normal overall QOL.[37–39] Undeniably, the lack of a comparative methodology decreases the reliability and reproducibility of such outcome reports. As pointed out in the recommendations of a consensus panel on laryngeal preservation led by Lefebvre and colleagues,[40] using a set of clinical end points and outcome criteria with a fairly high level of granularity as well as rigorous methodology for comparison of modalities would be desirable in the design of any clinical trial.[40] Other efforts such as a European proposal for a new partial laryngectomy nomenclature may contribute to foster more uniform and reproducible review of outcomes and coherent presentation of findings.[41] Regrettably, the study of the outcomes of transcervical partial laryngectomy, by virtue of the fact that it remains a rare option used only in a small number of centers, is certain to produce results with limited statistical power. This fact does not mean that the existing plethora of small series reports with valuable expert opinion should be discounted, particularly if the findings are consistent between various investigators.

Deglutition is one frequent source of apprehension when contemplating partial laryngectomy. SCPL routinely results in some degree of long-term trace aspiration once the patient resumes full oral diet, but this does not necessarily translate into significantly morbid aspiration events and is well tolerated by most patients after a period of adaptation.[42] Castro and colleagues[43] found that with proper patient selection, dysphagia scores remained excellent after SCPL and comparable to those observed after chemoradiation.

Another common focus of criticism of partial laryngectomy, and SCPL in particular, lies in deterioration of voice quality. Indeed, a review of objective voice quality indicators clearly favored TL and rehabilitation with tracheoesophageal prosthesis over SCPL.[44] This argument is often used by detractors of partial laryngectomy with the underlying claim that the presumably greater swallowing and phonatory function after TL should suffice to justify choosing it systematically over partial laryngectomy alternatives.

In fact, a more realistic and balanced perspective is warranted. While voice quality and swallowing function are undeniable elements of patient satisfaction, they represent merely a fraction of a vast QOL ensemble that is difficult to conceptualize and quantify. Leaving aside specific functional characterizations, higher-order QOL measurements should be viewed as key items of treatment outcome expectations.

Schindler and colleagues[38] recognized that despite resulting in poorer voice quality than TL, partial laryngectomy produced similar voice-related QOL. Other investigators observed greater overall QOL after partial laryngectomy compared with TL, including Weinstein and colleagues,[32] who found SCPL to produce superior QOL.[45]

As previously discussed, the presence of a permanent stoma can have a dramatic impact on QOL, illustrated by lower QOL scores after TL than after partial laryngectomy.[46] Partial laryngectomy appeared in one report to have the lowest psychosocial impact of the most commonly used modalities,[47] and SCPL was even found to result in almost normal biopsychosocial integration in a given patient population.[48]

Certain factors were found to limit the potential for QOL preservation after partial laryngectomy: SCPL with cricohyoidoepiglottopexy generally produces excellent QOL, but the rare scenario of inability to decannulate or comorbid association of radiotherapy or cervical lymphadenectomy seem to affect QOL scores negatively.[49] Nonetheless, salvage partial laryngectomy was noted to have acceptable functional—and oncologic—outcomes in carefully selected patients with stage I or II laryngeal disease not responding to definitive radiotherapy, making it a useful alternative to TL.[50]

Finally, some promising recent advances and ingenuous modifications of the surgical technique may allow for future expansion of the possibilities offered by partial laryngectomy. These efforts have resulted in improved voice quality, swallowing function, and decannulation time.[51–54] An overview of the general pros and cons of conservation laryngeal surgery is presented in **Table 1**.

ADVANCED AND RECURRENT LARYNGEAL CARCINOMA

The primary intricacy of conservation laryngeal surgery resides in adequate patient selection. Increasing complexity of patient selection is to be anticipated with an ongoing evolution of the open partial laryngectomy paradigm. For instance, it is commonly accepted that transcervical partial laryngectomy techniques are no longer appropriate in the routine management of early malignancies, in the manner they used to be until the end of the past century. The next conservation surgery frontiers to be explored lie in advanced laryngeal lesions and recurrent or persistent disease that has failed to respond to prior therapy, surgical or not.

Olthoff and colleagues[55] identified TLM as a modality that can be incorporated into existing algorithms and found that, in combination with adjuvant radiotherapy, TLM was a reasonable alternative in the management of advanced laryngeal cancer, with satisfactory rates of laryngeal preservation and QOL scores in spite of some expected functional morbidity.

Table 1 Summary of conservation laryngeal surgery attributes	
Advantages	**Disadvantages**
• Single intervention; revision partial resection often still feasible if needed • No permanent stoma • Favorable long-term/delayed morbidity profile • Total laryngectomy and nonsurgical modalities can be spared for ultimate control of persistent or recurrent disease • Accurate pathologic staging • Lower cost compared with radiation therapy	• Possible need for revision and multiple procedures • Histologic upstaging or adverse features may warrant adjuvant treatment • Specialized training and experience requirement • Possibly longer posttreatment interval before functional stabilization

In T3N0 disease of the glottis, Sessions and colleagues[31] noted open partial laryngectomy to generate results equivalent to definitive radiotherapy in terms of survival, voice quality, and permanent tracheotomy or stoma retention rates. As suggested previously, SCPL has excellent outcomes as the primary treatment modality of appropriately selected stage III and IV laryngeal cancer[30] and definitely deserves to be considered as a salvage option in situations usually leading to radical resection, as its rates of local control, decannulation, and preservation of functional voice and swallowing remain excellent even when performed after primary radiation therapy.[50,56,57]

SUMMARY

Although minimally invasive surgical approaches have considerably changed the landscape of laryngeal cancer management, time-honored conservation surgery techniques deserve to maintain a role in specific circumstances and may constitute an emerging alternative to total laryngectomy or radiation in advanced and recurrent laryngeal cancer.

The management of laryngeal cancer is a task of great complexity when one attempts to reconcile the best possible oncologic outcomes with optimized posttreatment function levels. The range of treatment approaches available and the variability of their respective long-term sequelae constitute infinite quandaries. The understanding of QOL not only as a summative, but also as an independent factor of patient satisfaction, is essential and has to be fully incorporated into the multidisciplinary treatment planning process.

REFERENCES

1. Demez PH, Moreau PR. Perception of head and neck cancer quality of life within the medical world: a multicultural study. Head Neck 2009;31:1056–67.
2. McNeil BJ, Weichselbaum R, Pauker SG. Speech and survival: tradeoffs between quality and quantity of life in laryngeal cancer. N Engl J Med 1981;305:982–7.
3. Bindewald J, Oeken J, Wollbrueck D, et al. Quality of life correlates after surgery for laryngeal carcinoma. Laryngoscope 2007;117:1770–6.
4. Moor JW, Rafferty A, Sood S. Can laryngectomees smell? Considerations regarding olfactory rehabilitation following total laryngectomy. J Laryngol Otol 2010;124:361–5.
5. Babin E, Blanchard D, Hitier M. Management of total laryngectomy patients over time: from the consultation announcing the diagnosis to long term follow-up. Eur Arch Otorhinolaryngol 2011;268:1407–19.
6. Babin E, Edy E, Bequignon A, et al. Personal and social identity transformations that occur over time among patients with total laryngectomy. J Otolaryngol Head Neck Surg 2008;37:495–501 [in French].
7. Lefebvre JL. The impact of a total laryngectomy on the patients' quality of life. Eur Arch Otorhinolaryngol 2011;268:1397–8.
8. Mallis A, Goumas PD, Mastronikolis NS, et al. Factors influencing quality of life after total laryngectomy: a study of 92 patients. Eur Rev Med Pharmacol Sci 2011;15:937–42.
9. DeSanto LW, Olsen KD, Perry WC, et al. Quality of life after surgical treatment of cancer of the larynx. Ann Otol Rhinol Laryngol 1995;104:763–9.
10. Potter CP, Birchall MA. Laryngectomees' views on laryngeal transplantation. Transpl Int 1998;11:433–8.
11. Induction chemotherapy plus radiation compared with surgery plus radiation in patients with advanced laryngeal cancer. The Department of Veterans Affairs Laryngeal Cancer Study Group. N Engl J Med 1991;324:1685–90.

12. American Society of Clinical Oncology, Pfister DG, Laurie SA, et al. American Society of Clinical Oncology clinical practice guideline for the use of larynx-preservation strategies in the treatment of laryngeal cancer. J Clin Oncol 2006; 24:3693–704.
13. Vilaseca I, Ballesteros F, Martinez-Vidal BM, et al. Quality of life after transoral laser microresection of laryngeal cancer: a longitudinal study. J Surg Oncol 2013;108:52–6.
14. Robertson SM, Yeo JC, Dunnet C, et al. Voice, swallowing, and quality of life after total laryngectomy: results of the west of Scotland laryngectomy audit. Head Neck 2012;34:59–65.
15. Steiner W. Results of curative laser microsurgery of laryngeal carcinomas. Am J Otolaryngol 1993;14:116–21.
16. Luo CM, Fang TJ, Lin CY, et al. Transoral laser microsurgery elevates fundamental frequency in early glottic cancer. J Voice 2012;26:596–601.
17. Oridate N, Homma A, Suzuki S, et al. Voice-related quality of life after treatment of laryngeal cancer. Arch Otolaryngol Head Neck Surg 2009;135:363–8.
18. Chu PY, Hsu YB, Lee TL, et al. Longitudinal analysis of voice quality in patients with early glottic cancer after transoral laser microsurgery. Head Neck 2012;34:1294–8.
19. Cohen SM, Garrett CG, Dupont WD, et al. Voice-related quality of life in T1 glottic cancer: irradiation versus endoscopic excision. Ann Otol Rhinol Laryngol 2006; 115:581–6.
20. Osborn HA, Hu A, Venkatesan V, et al. Comparison of endoscopic laser resection versus radiation therapy for the treatment of early glottic carcinoma. J Otolaryngol Head Neck Surg 2011;40:200–4.
21. Spielmann PM, Majumdar S, Morton RP. Quality of life and functional outcomes in the management of early glottic carcinoma: a systematic review of studies comparing radiotherapy and transoral laser microsurgery. Clin Otolaryngol 2010;35:373–82.
22. van Loon Y, Sjogren EV, Langeveld TP, et al. Functional outcomes after radiotherapy or laser surgery in early glottic carcinoma: a systematic review. Head Neck 2012;34:1179–89.
23. Ansarin M, Cattaneo A, Santoro L, et al. Laser surgery of early glottic cancer in elderly. Acta Otorhinolaryngol Ital 2010;30:169.
24. Phillips TJ, Sader C, Brown T, et al. Transoral laser microsurgery versus radiation therapy for early glottic cancer in Canada: cost analysis. J Otolaryngol Head Neck Surg 2009;38:619–23.
25. Silver CE, Beitler JJ, Shaha AR, et al. Current trends in initial management of laryngeal cancer: the declining use of open surgery. Eur Arch Otorhinolaryngol 2009;266:1333–52.
26. Olsen KD. Reexamining the treatment of advanced laryngeal cancer. Head Neck 2010;32:1–7.
27. Forastiere AA. Larynx preservation and survival trends: should there be concern? Head Neck 2010;32:14–7.
28. Wolf GT. Reexamining the treatment of advanced laryngeal cancer: the VA laryngeal cancer study revisited. Head Neck 2010;32:7–14.
29. Makeieff M, de la Breteque A, Guerrier B, et al. Voice handicap evaluation after supracricoid partial laryngectomy. Laryngoscope 2009;119:746–50.
30. Laudadio P, Presutti L, Dall'olio D, et al. Supracricoid laryngectomies: long-term oncological and functional results. Acta Otolaryngol 2006;126:640–9.
31. Sessions DG, Lenox J, Spector GJ, et al. Management of T3N0M0 glottic carcinoma: therapeutic outcomes. Laryngoscope 2002;112:1281–8.

32. Weinstein GS, El-Sawy MM, Ruiz C, et al. Laryngeal preservation with supracricoid partial laryngectomy results in improved quality of life when compared with total laryngectomy. Laryngoscope 2001;111:191–9.

33. Bussu F, Paludetti G, Almadori G, et al. Comparison of total laryngectomy with surgical (cricohyoidopexy) and nonsurgical organ-preservation modalities in advanced laryngeal squamous cell carcinomas: A multicenter retrospective analysis. Head Neck 2013;35:554–61.

34. Qian W, Zhu G, Wang Y, et al. Multi-modality management for loco-regionally advanced laryngeal and hypopharyngeal cancer: balancing the benefit of efficacy and functional preservation. Med Oncol 2014;31:178.

35. Portas JG, Queija Ddos S, Arine LP, et al. Voice and swallowing disorders: functional results and quality of life following supracricoid laryngectomy with cricohyoidoepiglottopexy. Ear Nose Throat J 2009;88:E23–30.

36. Saito K, Araki K, Ogawa K, et al. Laryngeal function after supracricoid laryngectomy. Otolaryngol Head Neck Surg 2009;140:487–92.

37. Crosetti E, Garofalo P, Bosio C, et al. How the operated larynx ages. Acta Otorhinolaryngol Ital 2014;34:19–28.

38. Schindler A, Favero E, Nudo S, et al. Long-term voice and swallowing modifications after supracricoid laryngectomy: objective, subjective, and self-assessment data. Am J Otolaryngol 2006;27:378–83.

39. Topaloglu I, Salturk Z, Atar Y, et al. Evaluation of voice quality after supraglottic laryngectomy. Otolaryngol Head Neck Surg 2014;151:1003–7.

40. Lefebvre JL, Ang KK, Larynx Preservation Consensus Panel. Larynx preservation clinical trial design: key issues and recommendations–a consensus panel summary. Head Neck 2009;31:429–41.

41. Rizzotto G, Crosetti E, Lucioni M, et al. Subtotal laryngectomy: outcomes of 469 patients and proposal of a comprehensive and simplified classification of surgical procedures. Eur Arch Otorhinolaryngol 2012;269:1635–46.

42. Webster KT, Samlan RA, Jones B, et al. Supracricoid partial laryngectomy: swallowing, voice, and speech outcomes. Ann Otol Rhinol Laryngol 2010;119: 10–6.

43. Castro A, Sanchez-Cuadrado I, Bernaldez R, et al. Laryngeal function preservation following supracricoid partial laryngectomy. Head Neck 2012;34:162–7.

44. Torrejano G, Guimaraes I. Voice quality after supracricoid laryngectomy and total laryngectomy with insertion of voice prosthesis. J Voice 2009;23:240–6.

45. Braz DS, Ribas MM, Dedivitis RA, et al. Quality of life and depression in patients undergoing total and partial laryngectomy. Clinics (Sao Paulo) 2005;60:135–42.

46. Ozturk A, Mollaoglu M. Determination of problems in patients with post-laryngectomy. Scand J Psychol 2013;54:107–11.

47. de Maddalena H, Pfrang H, Schohe R, et al. Speech intelligibility and psychosocial adaptation in various voice rehabilitation methods following laryngectomy. Laryngorhinootologie 1991;70:562–7 [in German].

48. Luna-Ortiz K, Nunz-Valencia ER, Tamez-Velarde M, et al. Quality of life and functional evaluation after supracricoid partial laryngectomy with cricohyoidoepiglottopexy in Mexican patients. J Laryngol Otol 2004;118:284–8.

49. Marquez Moyano JA, Sanchez Gutierrez R, Roldan Nogueras J, et al. Assessment of quality of life in patients treated by supracricoid partial laryngectomy with cricohyoidoepiglottopexy (CHEP). Acta Otorrinolaringol Esp 2004;55: 409–14 [in Spanish].

50. Philippe Y, Espitalier F, Durand N, et al. Partial laryngectomy as salvage surgery after radiotherapy: oncological and functional outcomes and impact on quality of

life. A retrospective study of 20 cases. Eur Ann Otorhinolaryngol Head Neck Dis 2014;131:15–9.

51. Allegra E, Lombardo N, La Boria A, et al. Quality of voice evaluation in patients treated by supracricoid laryngectomy and modified supracricoid laryngectomy. Otolaryngol Head Neck Surg 2011;145:789–95.

52. Maoxiao Y, Renyu L. Long-term outcomes of supracricoid partial laryngectomy with cricohyoidoepiglottopexy and its modified version. Saudi Med J 2013;34:282–7.

53. So YK, Yun YS, Baek CH, et al. Speech outcome of supracricoid partial laryngectomy: comparison with total laryngectomy and anatomic considerations. Otolaryngol Head Neck Surg 2009;141:770–5.

54. Yu Y, Wang XL, Xu ZG, et al. Laryngeal reconstruction with a sternohyoid muscle flap after supracricoid laryngectomy: postoperative respiratory and swallowing evaluation. Otolaryngol Head Neck Surg 2014;151:824–9.

55. Olthoff A, Ewen A, Wolff HA, et al. Organ function and quality of life after transoral laser microsurgery and adjuvant radiotherapy for locally advanced laryngeal cancer. Strahlenther Onkol 2009;185:303–9.

56. Marioni G, Marchese-Ragona R, Pastore A, et al. The role of supracricoid laryngectomy for glottic carcinoma recurrence after radiotherapy failure: a critical review. Acta Otolaryngol 2006;126:1245–51.

57. Motamed M, Laccourreye O, Bradley PJ. Salvage conservation laryngeal surgery after irradiation failure for early laryngeal cancer. Laryngoscope 2006;116:451–5.

Salvage Conservation Laryngeal Surgery After Radiation Therapy Failure

Michelle Mizhi Chen, MD[a], F. Christopher Holsinger, MD[b],*,
Ollivier Laccourreye, MD[c]

KEYWORDS

- Conservation laryngeal surgery • Larynx • Radiation • Salvage
- Supracricoid • Laser

KEY POINTS

- Many patients with recurrent tumors after radiation therapy (RT) with or without chemotherapy usually require total laryngectomy because of their advanced stage and functional decline.
- Radiorecurrent disease often presents with submucosal multifocal disease that is clinically understaged more than half the time.
- Patients undergoing salvage conservation laryngeal surgery (CLS) should be counseled about a substantially longer recovery than patients undergoing CLS as the primary therapy.
- Preoperative evaluation and postoperative rehabilitation with a speech language pathologist is critical for recovery after salvage CLS.
- Open CLS provides better oncologic outcomes for patients in the salvage setting, but transoral laser microsurgery (TLM) is associated with a shorter recovery and does not require an extensive rehabilitation process; however, TLM may require more than one procedure to achieve local control and has a lower rate of laryngeal preservation than supracricoid partial laryngectomy (SCPL).

INTRODUCTION

The incidence of larynx cancer in the United States for the year 2014 was estimated to be 12,630 cases, accounting for 3610 deaths, with a male/female ratio of 4:1.[1] Despite improvements in diagnostic and therapeutic techniques, the overall survival rate has not improved substantially during the past 25 years.[2]

[a] Division of Head and Neck Surgery, Department of Otolaryngology – Head and Neck Surgery, Stanford University, 801 Welch Road, Palo Alto, CA 94305-5820, USA; [b] Head and Neck Oncology Program, Division of Head and Neck Surgery, Department of Otolaryngology – Head and Neck Surgery, Stanford University, 875 Blake Wilbur Drive, Palo Alto, CA 94305-5820, USA; [c] Department of Otorhinolaryngology – Head and Neck Surgery, University Paris Descartes Sorbonne Paris Cité, Hôpital Européen Georges Pompidou, Assistance Publique – Hôpitaux de Paris, 20 rue Leblanc, Paris 70015, France
* Corresponding author.
E-mail address: holsinger@stanford.edu

Otolaryngol Clin N Am 48 (2015) 667–675
http://dx.doi.org/10.1016/j.otc.2015.04.011
0030-6665/15/$ – see front matter © 2015 Elsevier Inc. All rights reserved.

WHAT IS CONSERVATION LARYNGEAL SURGERY?

CLS[3] encompasses open surgical techniques such as laryngofissure with cordectomy and SCPLs; it also includes transoral endoscopic head and neck surgical techniques.[4] The cornerstone of CLS rests on these fundamental principles that optimize both oncologic and functional outcomes. The surgeon should consider CLS when the proposed surgery should have a high probability of achieving local control in the larynx and preserve at least 1 cricoarytenoid unit, which serves as the basic functional unit of the larynx. The cricoarytenoid unit includes 1 functioning arytenoid, an intact cricoid cartilage, associated laryngeal musculature, and corresponding innervation by the superior and recurrent laryngeal nerves. The conservation laryngeal surgeon must have carefully examined the extent of the patient's tumor to provide the patient with a high probability of completing the resection without requiring total laryngectomy. The conservation laryngeal surgeon must also understand that the resection of normal tissue may be necessary to achieve consistent functional outcomes. Finally, the patient and surgeon must understand and accept that a successful functional outcome after CLS following RT may take much longer to achieve than after primary CLS.

Laryngofissure with cordectomy is best suited for small, mid–vocal fold lesions not reaching the anterior commissure or the vocal process with no impairment of vocal fold mobility in patients in whom endoscopic exposure is inadequate. This approach involves splitting of the thyroid cartilage to gain access to the endolarynx and excise the affected vocal fold.[5] Although this procedure was previously characterized by the need for a perioperative tracheotomy,[6] Muscatello and colleagues[7] reported a series of 33 cases in which no tracheotomies were needed. In this cohort, the local control rate was 100%, the 5-year survival rate was 97%, and the laryngeal preservation rate was 100%. Danilidis and colleagues[8] observed similar results in a cohort of 94 patients with a 5-year survival rate of 93% but acknowledged that the survival rates were significantly poorer in patients who were treated with a laryngofissure and cordectomy for local recurrence after RT. Only 2 of the 5 patients treated with a salvage procedure survived for more than 5 years; the remainder died from another recurrence.[8]

Vertical partial laryngectomy (VPL) or vertical hemilaryngectomy entails extending a laryngofissure with cordectomy to include resection of the corresponding thyroid ala with the affected vocal fold, sparing the ipsilateral arytenoid and, if needed, the anterior commissure or the anterior one-third of the contralateral vocal fold. For T1 lesions treated with VPL, local control rates are 89% to 100%. Involvement of the anterior commissure decreases local control; one study reported that anterior commissure involvement decreased local control from 93% to 75%.[9] The same study found that local recurrence decreased the 10-year survival rate from 63% to 31%.[9] T2 tumors treated with VPL have local control rates of 74% to 86%. One meta-analysis review found better rates of local control in select patients without impairment of vocal fold immobility or significant extension to the subglottis or supraglottis.[10] VPL as salvage surgery for early-stage glottic cancers that recur after RT has been shown to have rates of local control ranging from 55% to 100%, without significantly different functional outcomes from those who had VPL as the primary surgery.[11–13] Laccourreye and colleagues[14] observed a 78.1% laryngeal preservation rate for VPL in the salvage setting, strictly in patients in whom the tumor has not enlarged. In a study comparing 21 patients who had prior RT with 41 previously untreated patients, Lydiatt and colleagues[11] determined that there was no significant difference in 5-year survival (79% vs 95%, P = NS), although survival was clearly better when CLS was performed in previously untreated patients. Moreover, functional outcomes, such as time to tracheotomy decannulation and swallowing function at the time of discharge, were not significantly different between the irradiated group and the previously untreated group.[11]

In a supraglottic laryngectomy (SGL), or horizontal partial laryngectomy, the larynx is resected between the pre-epiglottic space and the ventricles, with preservation of both true vocal folds, both arytenoids, and the hyoid bone. Extended procedures may include resection of the tongue base, arytenoids, aryepiglottic fold, or superior medial pyriform wall. Contraindications to SGL are involvement of the glottis, thyroid or cricoid cartilage invasion, tongue base involvement within 1 cm of the circumvallate papillae, major pre-epiglottic space invasion, and deep musculature involvement in the tongue base.[5] Local control rates after SGL are 92% to 100% for T1 lesions and 85% to 100% for T2 tumors. DeSanto and colleagues[15] underscored that, although 80% (24 of 30) of patients with supraglottic carcinoma who underwent RT and failed would have been theoretically amenable to SGL before RT, only 30% (9 of 30) underwent CLS for failure after RT. Sørensen and colleagues[16] noted poor oncologic and functional results after SGL for RT failure and advocated total laryngectomy in these patients. Yiotakis and colleagues[13] examined 9 patients who had SGL after RT failure and found that 4 of the 9 had recurrent disease within 2 years and the overall survival rate was 67%.

SCPLs[17] involve the resection of both true and false vocal folds, the thyroid cartilage, both paraglottic spaces, and 1 partial or full arytenoid. The epiglottis and pre-epiglottic space may or may not be included according to the tumor origin and extent. This procedure is reconstructed with either a cricohyoidoepiglottopexy in glottis cancer or a cricohyoidopexy in supraglottic and transglottic ones. SCPLs are used for T1b and T2 carcinomas and selected T3 cancer (pre-epiglottic space invasion, thyroid cartilage, and true vocal cord fixation). Contraindications to SCPL include arytenoid cartilage fixation, invasion of the cricoid or posterior commissure, subglottic extension to level of the cricoid, and extension to or beyond the outer perichondrium of the thyroid cartilage.[10] For T1 and T2 lesions, the 5-year actuarial estimate of local control is as high as 98%[18]; another study reported rates of 96% and 91% for T1 and T2 tumors, respectively.[19] Overall, local control rates range from 87% to 98%, and overall 5-year actuarial estimates of survival range from 73% to 79%, with disease-specific survival estimated at 94%.[20] The mortality rate for SCPL is low (1%–2%), with a 9.6% to 11% postoperative morbidity rate. Laccourreye and colleagues[21] evaluated the role of SCPLs as a salvage technique after failed laryngeal RT in 12 cases and determined a 3-year actuarial survival and local control rate of 83%. The time to tracheotomy decannulation was twice as long in these patients (average of 15 days) than in cases of SCPLs in patients who have not received RT, likely due to significant postoperative edema in the arytenoid cartilages and the delayed healing present in irradiated tissues.[21] A more recent multi-institutional study by Pellini and colleagues[22] of 78 patients who received SCPLs in the salvage setting observed 3- and 5-year disease-free survival rates of 96% and 3- and 5-year overall survival rates of 85% and 82%, respectively. Within 1 year, most cases were able to be decannulated and achieve adequate swallowing (97%).[22] Laryngeal preservation rates for SCPL in the salvage setting have been shown to be around 90%.[23]

TLM is well established in the primary management of early-stage larynx cancer.[24] The 5-year disease-free survival rate in early-stage glottic cancer treated primarily by TLM is 81% to 93%.[25] However, the usage of TLM for recurrent larynx cancer often requires repeat surgery. In patients with recurrent disease after RT, Steiner and colleagues[26] reported that only 38% achieved local control after the first TLM and 6% of patients required 4 procedures. A meta-analysis reported that the pooled outcome for local control in radio recurrent disease with the first TLM is 56.9% and 63.8% with repeat TLM.[27] The pooled laryngeal preservation rate was 72.3%.[27] Even when repeat TLM is taken into account, the oncologic outcomes of TLM for recurrent laryngeal cancer are inferior to those of open CLS techniques. The postoperative complication rate and recovery rate are less in TLM compared with open CLS techniques. Steiner and colleagues[26] observed that 9% had glottic synechia and 3% had laryngeal stenosis after repeated TLM procedures. The average hospital stay was 9 days.[26]

STRATEGY OF CONSERVATION LARYNGEAL SURGERY AFTER RADIATION THERAPY FAILURE: WHEN, FOR WHICH TUMORS, AND WHY?

Local failure rates for RT for early-stage larynx cancer have been estimated to be 5% to 10% for T1 lesions and 20% to 40% for T2 lesions.[28] RT failures in limited disease are often caused by errors in initial staging based on clinical criteria; hence, it is important to perform careful staging after a thorough endoscopic examination aided by computed tomographic (CT) findings. It is important to understand the pattern and spread of recurrent early larynx cancer to select patients who would be best suited for salvage CLS. Although most primary larynx cancers demonstrate concentric tumor growth (77%), only a fifth of recurrent cancers presented in that manner (19%).[29] Recurrent larynx cancer more commonly presents with multifocal tumor nests (86%), dissociated tumor cells (76%), and perineural spread (81%).[29] Viani and colleagues[30] observed that in patients with T1–3N0 glottic cancer, more than 80% of the recurrent tumors were pT3–4. De Vincentiis and colleagues[31] reviewed 68 patients with recurrent larynx cancer who underwent salvage by either total laryngectomy or SCPL and determined that the method of salvage was not associated with overall survival but positive margins were independently associated with decreased survival (hazard ratio, 11.3; $P = .02$). Toma and colleagues[32] observed that patients with margins less than 1 mm had significantly higher recurrence rates after salvage CLS than those with margins of 1 mm or more.

Radiation treatment induces inflammatory and fibrotic changes in tissue that makes the clinical assessment of the extent of recurrent disease more difficult because of posttherapeutic edema, erythema, and changes in laryngeal mobilities.[33] Consequently, the clinical assessment of recurrence by endoscopic examination and imaging has a diagnostic accuracy of 38%, with 10% of the tumors overstaged and 52% understaged.[29] Diagnosis of recurrent disease is based on clinical suspicion, follow-up CT findings, and direct endoscopy with biopsy, although caution should be maintained when taking a biopsy from a post-RT larynx because of the risk of chondritis. All this often leads to late discovery of the recurrence, leaving many patients who are eligible for surgical salvage needing to undergo total laryngectomy.[15,34]

Som[35] was the first to publish results on CLS as salvage therapy after RT in 1951. More recently, Ganly and colleagues[28] noted that local control rates for salvage total laryngectomy were 65% to 85% for T1 and T2 glottic tumors, whereas local control rates for salvage CLS range from 66% to 96%. Although CLS can be an effective salvage therapy,

most patients with recurrent or persistent disease after RT end up with a total laryngectomy because they often present with advanced disease. Because recurrent tumors can
be unpredictable and have adverse features, patients should be informed about the
possible need for a total laryngectomy during preoperative planning for CLS. In 1990,
Shah and colleagues[36] recommended excluding patients from CLS if recurrent disease
extends beyond the original site. One year later, Lavey and Calcaterra[12] stated, after a review of the literature, that vertical hemilaryngectomy should be contraindicated in the RT
failure case if the tumor involved the arytenoids, there was more than 10 mm of subglottic
extension anteriorly and 5 mm posteriorly, and cartilage invasion into the thyroid or the
cricoid was demonstrated to be present. For supraglottic cancer, Shaw[37] stated that
SGL is contraindicated in the post-RT failure setting unless the primary tumor was small,
the recurrence was located anteriorly, and the carcinoma never involved the anterior
commissure. However, these indications were made at a time when quality CT laryngeal
scan evaluation was not widely diffused and only VPL and SGPL were the CLS techniques
available because neither TLM nor SCPL was widely known and used. Institutional
studies have demonstrated that 32% to 52% of patients with early-stage recurrent cancer after RT are candidates for salvage with CLS.[28,38–40]

Even in the N0 recurrent laryngeal cancer, prophylactic neck dissection should be
considered, although this procedure should be considered individually across the
laryngeal subsites. A retrospective review reported a 0% incidence of occult cervical
metastases with T1 and T2 glottic cancer.[41] Deganello and colleagues[23] examined 26
patients with N0 cancer with recurrent disease after RT managed with SCPLs and
determined a 19% rate of occult neck metastasis. All of the patients with occult
neck metastases had clinically T1 disease that was upstaged to T2–3, and the investigators suggested the use of ipsilateral elective neck dissections in these select patients. Supraglottic cancers present with a higher incidence of cervical metastasis;
up to 30% of patients with N0 cancer have occult lymph node metastases.[42] It is
therefore recommended that the levels II–IV of the neck be addressed bilaterally for
all supraglottic tumors, either surgically or with radiotherapy, whereas treatment of
the neck may not be indicated for early recurrent glottic cancer with N0 disease.
Yao and colleagues[43] observed a 20% rate of occult metastases in patients with
T3–T4 recurrent glottic cancer and in patients with supraglottic cancer and recommended bilateral elective neck dissections in these cohorts.

FUNCTIONAL REHABILITATION AFTER SALVAGE CONSERVATION LARYNGEAL SURGERY FOR RADIATION THERAPY FAILURE

The selection process for patients who are good candidates for CLS includes a preoperative assessment of pulmonary function and a willingness to participate in the
extensive rehabilitation process required postoperatively. Patients who undergo
CLS for recurrent disease have delayed time to decannulation and nasogastric
tube/percutaneous endoscopic gastrostomy (PEG) tube removal but are able to be
decannulated and achieve normal swallowing by 1 year at rates similar to those
who undergo CLS for primary disease.

Complications following CLS after previous RT include infection, bleeding, adhesions, cutaneous fistulae, stenosis, aspiration pneumonia, feeding tube or tracheotomy dependence, persistent and obstructive granulation tissue, and
tracheocutaneous fistulae. The incidence of postoperative morbidity correlates with
a previous history of irradiation, especially in the instances of local wound healing
complications such as laryngeal stenosis and rupture of the pexy in SCPL. The complication rate after salvage CLS is reported to be 19% to 28%, with a fistula rate of 8% to

19%.[28,44,45] An analysis of 150 patients who had CLS by Ganly and colleagues[46] demonstrated that prior RT was not associated with overall complications but was independently associated with local complications (relative risk of 13.2, $P = .004$). When comparing the results of patients who received SCPL as salvage surgery after RT with those who received SCPL as the primary surgery, there are slightly higher early (18.1% vs 10.5%) and late complication rates (17.9% vs 14.3%).[47] Mucosal edema generally persists for a longer time in irradiated tissue, resulting in a delay in decannulation for patients who have received RT previously, but the rates of decannulation at 1 year are similar between those who had SCPL as the primary surgery and those who received salvage surgery.[21,22,47] In a recent case series, Ganly and colleagues[28] analyzed 21 patients who had salvage CLS for early-stage larynx cancer and reported an overall postoperative complication rate of 19%, with the most common complications being local wound and fistula complications. In patients who received salvage total laryngectomy, the rate of fistula occurrence was 15% in patients who had prior RT and 30% in patients who had prior chemoradiation.[48] Thus, the postoperative complication rate is similar between salvage CLS and salvage total laryngectomy.

SUMMARY

Forty years after the Centennial Conference on Laryngeal Cancer in Toronto in 1974,[49] the selection criteria and treatment algorithm to identify patients suitable for salvage CLS in recurrent laryngeal cancer have continued to evolve and improve.[49] In light of many improvements in surgical technique, innovative novel procedures, as well as new technology for pathology, imaging, and rehabilitation, the authors summarize 4 criteria for surgeons to consider when evaluating patients with recurrent or persistence tumor after treatment with RT for CLS.

1. Identify any contraindication to CLS. A surgeon should not consider laryngeal-preservation surgery if the following features are noted: (1) fixation of the arytenoid cartilage, (2) invasion of the posterior commissure, (3) subglottic extension of more than 5 mm posteriorly and 5 to 10 mm anteriorly, and (4) cricoid cartilage invasion and major thyroid cartilage invasion (T4).[28,40] In such cases, the patient should be offered a salvage total laryngectomy because the risk for local failure is too high regardless of the CLS technique that is used.
2. Determine the surgical technique that will result in the best chances for local control. TLM, VPL, and SGPL may be used when the recurrent disease does not extend beyond the original site and the larynx is mobile. However, when the recurrent tumor extends beyond its original site, results in impaired motion or fixation of the vocal cord, and/or presents with pre-epiglottic space or thyroid cartilage invasion, then SCPLs should be strongly advocated. In such cases, SCPLs offer wider mucosal and muscular margins while resulting in removal of the thyroid cartilage.
3. Estimate functional outcomes after salvage SCPLs when compared with salvage TLM, VPL, or SGPL, with the need for careful analysis of the patient's comorbidities and capacity to undergo a lengthy postoperative rehabilitation process.
4. Survey and assess for synchronous regional lymphatic and/or systemic disease relapse.[30]

Although the spectrum of salvage CLS has expanded during the past 25 years, many patients in whom the condition recurs after RT are not amenable to CLS. Using the criteria discussed earlier, the surgeon can still preserve the larynx and life in the appropriate selected patient. Yet, perhaps as importantly, the difficulty of successfully performing CLS as salvage therapy should inform patient decision making and multidisciplinary treatment planning when first-line treatment is selected. A more robust discussion of surgical options, as well as up-front RT, should be considered in every head and neck multidisciplinary tumor board.

REFERENCES

1. Siegel R, Ma J, Zou Z, et al. Cancer statistics, 2014. CA Cancer J Clin 2014;64: 9–29.
2. Jemal A, Siegel R, Ward E, et al. Cancer Statistics, 2008. CA Cancer J Clin 2008; 58:71–96.
3. Ogura JH. Selection of patients for conservation surgery of the larynx and pharynx. Trans Am Acad Ophthalmol Otolaryngol 1972;76:741–51.
4. Holsinger F. Robotics and transoral endoscopic head and neck surgery. In: Harrison LB, Sessions RB, Kies MS, editors. Head and neck cancer: a multidisciplinary approach. Philadelphia (PA): Lippincott Williams & Wilkins; 2013. p. 143–52.
5. Daly JF, Kwok FN. Laryngofissure and cordectomy. Laryngoscope 1975;85: 1290–7.
6. Olsen KD, Thomas JV, Desanto LW, et al. Indications and results of cordectomy for early glottic carcinoma. Otolaryngol Head Neck Surg 1993;108:277–82.
7. Muscatello L, Laccourreye O, Biacabe B, et al. Laryngofissure and cordectomy for glottic carcinoma limited to the mid third of the mobile true vocal cord. Laryngoscope 1997;107:1507–10.
8. Danilidis J, Nikolaou A, Symeonidis V. Our experience in the surgical treatment of T1 carcinoma of the vocal cord. J Laryngol Otol 1990;104:222–4.
9. Laccourreye O, Weinstein G, Brasnu D, et al. Vertical partial laryngectomy: a critical analysis of local recurrence. Ann Otol Rhinol Laryngol 1991;100:68–71.
10. Tufano RP, Stafford EM. Organ preservation surgery for laryngeal cancer. Otolaryngol Clin North Am 2008;41:741–55.
11. Lydiatt WM, Shah JP, Lydiatt KM. Conservation surgery for recurrent carcinoma of the glottic larynx. Am J Surg 1996;172:662–4.
12. Lavey RS, Calcaterra TC. Partial laryngectomy for glottic cancer after high-dose radiotherapy. Am J Surg 1991;162:341–4.
13. Yiotakis J, Stavroulaki P, Nikolopoulos T, et al. Partial laryngectomy after irradiation failure. Otolaryngol Head Neck Surg 2003;128:200–9.
14. Laccourreye O, Laccourreye L, Garcia D, et al. Vertical partial laryngectomy versus supracricoid partial laryngectomy for selected carcinomas of the true vocal cord classified as T2N0. Ann Otol Rhinol Laryngol 2000;109:965–71.
15. Desanto LW, Lillie JC, Devine KD. Surgical salvage after radiation for laryngeal cancer. Laryngoscope 1976;86:649–57.
16. Sørensen H, Hansen HS, Thomsen KA. Partial laryngectomy following irradiation. Laryngoscope 1980;90:1344–9.
17. Holsinger FC, Laccourreye O, Weinstein GS, et al. Technical refinements in the supracricoid partial laryngectomy to optimize functional outcomes. J Am Coll Surg 2005;201:809–20.
18. Laccourreye O, Muscatello L, Laccourreye L, et al. Supracricoid partial laryngectomy with cricohyoidoepiglottopexy for "early" glottic carcinoma classified as T1-T2N0 invading the anterior commissure. Am J Otolaryngol 1997;18:385–90.
19. Kania R, Hans S, Garcia D, et al. Supracricoid hemilaryngopharyngectomy in patients with invasive squamous cell carcinoma of the pyriform sinus. Part II: incidence and consequences of local recurrence. Ann Otol Rhinol Laryngol 2005;114:95–104.

20. Karasalihoglu AR, Yagiz R, Tas A, et al. Supracricoid partial laryngectomy with cricohyoidopexy and cricohyoidoepiglottopexy: functional and oncological results. J Laryngol Otol 2004;118:671–5.
21. Laccourreye O, Weinstein G, Naudo P, et al. Supracricoid partial laryngectomy after failed laryngeal radiation therapy. Laryngoscope 1996;106:495–8.
22. Pellini R, Pichi B, Ruscito P, et al. Supracricoid partial laryngectomies after radiation failure: a multi-institutional series. Head Neck 2008;30:372–9.
23. Deganello A, Gallo O, De Cesare JM, et al. Supracricoid partial laryngectomy as salvage surgery for radiation therapy failure. Head Neck 2008;30:1064–71.
24. Steiner W. Results of curative laser microsurgery of laryngeal carcinomas. Am J Otolaryngol 1993;14:116–21.
25. Lee HS, Chun B-G, Kim SW, et al. Transoral laser microsurgery for early glottic cancer as one-stage single-modality therapy. Laryngoscope 2013;123:2670–4.
26. Steiner W, Vogt P, Ambrosch P, et al. Transoral carbon dioxide laser microsurgery for recurrent glottic carcinoma after radiotherapy. Head Neck 2004;26:477–84.
27. Ramakrishnan Y, Drinnan M, Kwong FNK, et al. Oncologic outcomes of transoral laser microsurgery for radiorecurrent laryngeal carcinoma: a systematic review and meta-analysis of English-language literature. Head Neck 2014;36:280–5.
28. Ganly I, Patel SG, Matsuo J, et al. Results of surgical salvage after failure of definitive radiation therapy for early-stage squamous cell carcinoma of the glottic larynx. Arch Otolaryngol Head Neck Surg 2006;132:59–66.
29. Zbären P, Nuyens M, Curschmann J, et al. Histologic characteristics and tumor spread of recurrent glottic carcinoma: analysis on whole-organ sections and comparison with tumor spread of primary glottic carcinomas. Head Neck 2007;29:26–32.
30. Viani L, Stell PM, Dalby JE. Recurrence after radiotherapy for glottic carcinoma. Cancer 1991;67:577–84.
31. De Vincentiis M, De Virgilio A, Bussu F, et al. Oncologic results of the surgical salvage of recurrent laryngeal squamous cell carcinoma in a multicentric retrospective series: emerging role of supracricoid partial laryngectomy. Head Neck 2015;37:84–91.
32. Toma M, Nibu K, Nakao K, et al. Partial laryngectomy to treat early glottic cancer after failure of radiation therapy. Arch Otolaryngol Head Neck Surg 2002;128:909–12.
33. Ward PH, Calcaterra TC, Kagan AR. The enigma of post-radiation edema and recurrent or residual carcinoma of the larynx. Laryngoscope 1975;85:522–9.
34. Skolnik EM, Martin L, Yee KF, et al. Radiation failures in cancer of the larynx. Ann Otol Rhinol Laryngol 1975;84:804–11.
35. Som ML. Limited surgery after failure of radiotherapy in the treatment of carcinoma of the larynx. Ann Otol Rhinol Laryngol 1951;60:695–703.
36. Shah JP, Loree TR, Kowalski L. Conservation surgery for radiation-failure carcinoma of the glottic larynx. Head Neck 1990;12:326–31.
37. Shaw HJ. Role of partial laryngectomy after irradiation in the treatment of laryngeal cancer: a view from the United Kingdom. Ann Otol Rhinol Laryngol 1991;100:268–73.
38. Holsinger FC, Funk E, Roberts DB, et al. Conservation laryngeal surgery versus total laryngectomy for radiation failure in laryngeal cancer. Head Neck 2006;28:779–84.
39. Rodríguez-Cuevas S, Labastida S, Gonzalez D, et al. Partial laryngectomy as salvage surgery for radiation failures in T1–T2 laryngeal cancer. Head Neck 1998;20:630–3.

40. Biller HF, Barnhill FR, Ogura JH, et al. Hemilaryngectomy following radiation failure for carcinoma of the vocal cords. Laryngoscope 1970;80:249–53.
41. Yang CY, Andersen PE, Everts EC, et al. Nodal disease in purely glottic carcinoma: is elective neck treatment worthwhile? Laryngoscope 1998;108:1006–8.
42. Hicks WL, Kollmorgen DR, Kuriakose MA, et al. Patterns of nodal metastasis and surgical management of the neck in supraglottic laryngeal carcinoma. Otolaryngol Head Neck Surg 1999;121:57–61.
43. Yao M, Roebuck JC, Holsinger FC, et al. Elective neck dissection during salvage laryngectomy. Am J Otolaryngol 2005;26:388–92.
44. Nibu K, Kamata S, Kawabata K, et al. Partial laryngectomy in the treatment of radiation-failure of early glottic carcinoma. Head Neck 1997;19:116–20.
45. Watters GW, Patel SG, Rhys-Evans PH. Partial laryngectomy for recurrent laryngeal carcinoma. Clin Otolaryngol Allied Sci 2000;25:146–52.
46. Ganly I, Patel SG, Matsuo J, et al. Analysis of postoperative complications of open partial laryngectomy. Head Neck 2009;31:338–45.
47. Naudo P, Laccourreye O, Weinstein G, et al. Complications and functional outcome after supracricoid partial laryngectomy with cricohyoidoepiglottopexy. Otolaryngol Head Neck Surg 1998;118:124–9.
48. Weber RS, Berkey BA, Forastiere A, et al. Outcome of salvage total laryngectomy following organ preservation therapy: the radiation therapy oncology group trial 91-11. Arch Otolaryngol Head Neck Surg 2003;129:44–9.
49. Workshop No. 6, Centennial Conference on Laryngeal Cancer, Toronto, 1974. Can J Otolaryngol 1975;4:392–458.

Transoral and Transcervical Surgical Innovations in the Treatment of Glottic Cancer

Steven M. Zeitels, MD

KEYWORDS

- Vocal cord cancer • Glottic cancer • Larynx cancer • Phonosurgery
- Phonomicrosurgery • Airway reconstruction • Voice outcome

KEY POINTS

- Fiber-based 532 nm potassium titanyl phosphate (KTP) laser treatment of early glottic cancer combines the selectivity and precision of microsurgery with discreet zonal nonionizing radiation (photoangiolysis) integrating the assets of both conventional surgery and radiotherapy.
- Early glottic cancer can be optimally managed oncologically and with regards to voice outcome by means of photoangiolysis using the 532 nm KTP laser.
- Early glottic cancer that invades both vocal cords can be removed in 2 (staged) procedures so as to preserve the anatomic architecture of the anterior commissure and thereby achieve a better voice result as compared to a single procedure.
- Radiotherapy can be preserved as an oncologic treatment option in over 90% of patients with early glottic cancer, so that this single-use cancer treatment can be preserved for metachronous larger lesions.
- Transplantation of cryopreserved aortic homograft can be used effectively to restore the airway caliber in wide-field partial laryngectomy defects for advanced glottic cancer that extends subglottically.

EARLY GLOTTIC CANCER
Background

Transoral endoscopic removal of glottic cancer was reported first in 1888 as a mirror-guided piecemeal resection approach.[1] Approximately 30 years later, Lynch reported a bimanual, direct, suspension laryngoscopic method[2,3] that was later enhanced by

Disclosures: This work was supported in part by the Voice Health Institute, The "V" Foundation, the Eugene B. Casey Foundation, and the National Philanthropic Trust.
The author has an equity interest in Endocraft LLC, which produced the Universal Modular Glottiscope, from which the microlaryngeal photographs were obtained.
Division of Laryngeal Surgery, Massachusetts General Hospital, Harvard Medical School, One Bowdoin Square, Boston, MA 02114, USA
E-mail address: zeitels.steven@mgh.harvard.edu

Otolaryngol Clin N Am 48 (2015) 677–685
http://dx.doi.org/10.1016/j.otc.2015.04.012
0030-6665/15/$ – see front matter
oto.theclinics.com

Abbreviation
KTP   Potassium titanyl phosphate

the magnification provided by the surgical microscope. In the late 1960s and early 1970s, Jako,[4,5] Strong,[6,7] and Vaughan[8,9] introduced a carbon dioxide laser that was coupled to the surgical microscope, which ultimately became the watershed innovation that facilitated widespread adoption of endolaryngeal cancer surgery. In recent years, fiber-based delivery systems have further enhanced this method by providing substantially better control of the operative field.

Given the long successful history of endoscopic treatment of early glottic cancer, there is no controversy about its feasibility and success. Unlike other sites of the upper aerodigestive tract, early glottic cancers (T1 and T2 tumors) rarely metastasize, which provides unique opportunities for staged treatment strategies. Furthermore, because the cure rate is extremely high for any surgical approach or radiotherapy, the key metric for success in today's communication-based society is predicated on the voice outcome. It is also important to preserve future treatment options.

Optimal voice preservation is improved by the surgeon's keen awareness of vocal physiology. This functional understanding provides insights into the voice impact of a spectrum of neoplastic lesions prior to treatment, subsequent to resection, and after phonosurgical reconstruction. The reconstructive strategies are designed to enhance aerodynamic glottal competency. In the overwhelming majority of patients treated for early glottic cancer, the primary sound source is the remaining phonatory mucosa that is not involved with the cancer. It is also valuable to maintain adequate mucous hydration, which is provided by the glands of the saccule. Therefore, avoiding ionizing radiation to normal-residual phonatory mucosa and the saccular glands is advantageous.

Noncancerous phonatory mucosa is driven into oscillation by preserving or re-establishing aerodynamic competency after the tumor is treated. This is achieved by

Minimizing soft tissue removal through extremely narrow margins

Preserving the architecture of the rima glottidis by means of metachronous treatment of each vocal fold and preserving the structure of the anterior commissure

Reconstructing the paraglottic compartment by means of transoral and/or transcervical medialization procedures if an extensive amount of vocal musculature has been removed[10–12]

Endoscopic Angiolytic Potassium Titanyl Phosphate Laser Treatment of Early Glottic Cancer

Approximately 8 years ago, the author abandoned carbon dioxide laser excision of early glottic cancer in favor of angiolytic laser involution of the disease in order to maximize preservation of glottal soft tissue. Angiolytic laser removal of early glottic cancer with ultranarrow margins was first published in a pilot study 6 years ago as an innovative surgical treatment strategy to better preserve vocal function.[13]

It is likely that this was the first demonstration of employing nonionizing radiation without chemical enhancement (eg, photosensitizing agents) to involute and treat cancer without resection or gross ablation. This approach combines elements of surgery and radiation to create a unique hybrid approach.

Considering that the 3 conventional cancer treatments (surgery, radiotherapy, cytotoxic chemotherapy) evolved from the primary basic sciences (biology, physics, chemistry) Folkman's conception of antiangiogenesis agents became the fourth cancer treatment.[14] However, these agents are used as an adjuvant with other conventional treatment modalities. Based on discussions with Dr J. Folkman (personal communication, 2007), photoangiolytic laser treatment of the glottis is likely the first single-modality organ cancer treatment, which capitalizes on his philosophy that tumors retain denser blood supply and microcirculation as compared with normal surrounding soft tissue.

Photoangiolytic treatment of aerodigestive tract cancer has been done primarily with the 532 nm green-light KTP laser. The author had introduced angiolytic lasers (585 nm pulsed-dye laser, 532 nm pulsed-KTP laser) to facilitate microflap resection of glottal dysplasia in the late 1990s. Then, photoangiolysis of the subepithelial microcirculation allowed for extremely precise microflap epithelial resection, preservation of histopathological architecture, and minimal collateral thermal damage to the perivascular superficial lamina propria (SLP).[15,16]

The promise of the angiolytic laser treatment of early glottic cancer was supported by concepts of aberrant neovascularity described by Jako and Kleinsasser **(Fig. 1)**[4] in 1966 and intralesional tumor angiogenesis **(Figs. 2 and 3)** established by Folkman shortly thereafter in 1971.[14]

During the past 8 years, over 200 glottic cancers have been treated by 532 nm KTP photoangiolysis, and results of a cohort with long-term follow-up were recently published.[17] In that investigation, 117 patients (T1a-71, T1b-11, T2-10 unilateral/25 bilateral) underwent KTP laser treatment of early glottic cancer with a minimum 3-year follow-up (average: 53 months). Disease control for T1 and T2 lesions was 96% (79/82) and 80% (28/35), respectively. All 10 recurrences were treated with radiotherapy. Fifty percent (5/10) were controlled with radiotherapy, and the other 5 patients died of disease. Larynx preservation and survival were achieved in 99% (81/82) of patients with T1 disease and 89% (31/35) of patients with T2 disease.

This investigation provided clear evidence that angiolytic KTP laser treatment of early glottic cancer with ultranarrow margins was an effective surgical treatment

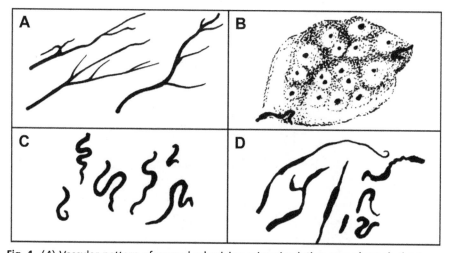

Fig. 1. (*A*) Vascular pattern of normal arborizing microcirculation seen through the transparent epithelium and within the superficial lamina propria of the phonatory mucosa. (*B*) Precancerous dysplasia of the epithelium obscures visualization of the subepithelial microcirculation. (*C, D*) Invasive carcinoma is comprised of aberrant disordered and dense microvasculature. (*From* Jako GJ, Kleinsasser O. Endolaryngeal micro-diagnosis and microsurgery. Reprint from the Annual Meeting of the American Medical Association. 1966.)

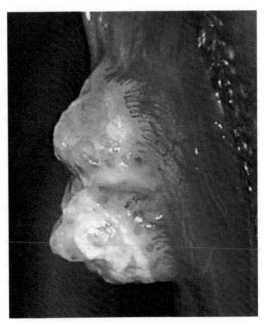

Fig. 2. Early vocal fold cancer demonstrating complex looping angiogenic microcirculation.

strategy. Radiotherapy was preserved as an oncologic option for future use in 94% of patients and effectively salvaged half of patients who failed endoscopic treatment.

The voice results that the author achieved with angiolytic KTP laser treatment[18] were superior to what could be achieved in the past with the CO_2 laser. This is especially so for those patients who have bilateral disease. Pretreatment and post-treatment voice outcome data were obtained for 92 patients (T1-64, T2-28) who underwent 532 nm KTP-laser treatment of early glottic cancer utilizing a design in which each patient essentially served as his or her own control. Evaluations included

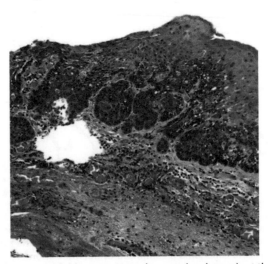

Fig. 3. Histology of a T1 vocal fold cancer. Note the vascular channels at the base of the nests of malignant epithelial cells and the ingrowth of vessels within the neoplasm.

objective measures (acoustic and aerodynamic) and patients' self-assessments of vocal function (voice-related quality of life, VRQOL). A series of mixed Analysis of variance with tumor stage and depth of invasion as the between-subject variables and time (before surgery vs after surgery) as the within variables was conducted for all vocal function measures.

There are several reasons for the improved voices, all of which can be explained by improvements in post-treatment aerodynamic competency of the glottis and/or enhanced phonatory mucosal pliability. Both were achieved through increased preservation of glottal soft tissue including noncancerous superficial lamina propria, the layer necessary for glottal vibration and optimal architecture of the rima glottidis.

Unlike prior microlaryngeal laser techniques that are used exclusively as a scalpel or indiscriminate ablating device (eg, CO_2, continuous-wave KTP, Thulium, Pleasanton CA), angiolytic lasers concentrate the energy within the dense aberrant angiogenic microcirculation of the tumors while not penetrating deeply into the normal soft tissue of the vocal fold. Thick tumors are vaporized in a continuous wave mode with simultaneous cooling until the interface with normal underlying soft tissue. The interface is treated in a pulsed mode, and frozen section margins are obtained from the patient to establish that the tumor has been removed.

By confining the pulse-width to no more than 15 milliseconds, the angiolytic laser induces selective heating of the lesions' intralesional/subepithelial microcirculation. This minimizes thermal trauma and fibrosis of the extralesional underlying normal glottal soft-tissue, thereby optimally preserving vocal fold soft tissue necessary for phonatory vibration. Photoangiolytic pulsed-laser treatment of early glottic cancer has the capability of preserving paraglottic space soft tissue in deeper neoplasms as well as mucosal SLP in more superficial tumors (**Fig. 4**).

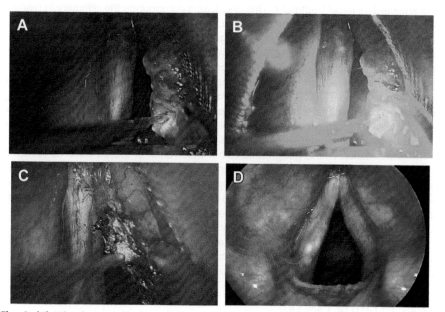

Fig. 4. (*A*) Microlaryngoscopic examination of a right vocal fold cancer with a 4 mm KTP laser fiber is directed at the tumor. (*B*) A 15 millisecond pulse of green light is absorbed at the intralesional microcirculation. (*C*) Toward the end of the cancer treatment. (*D*) Office laryngoscopic examination after healing—the patient is over 4 years without recurrence.

Cancer involvement of the anterior commissure tendon and/or the arytenoid cartilage is not a contraindication to this technique if adequate laryngoscopic exposure can be obtained. Thyroid cartilage invasion is a contraindication to this approach and requires transcervical removal of the thyroid lamina. To preserve the architecture of the anterior commissure, it is common to remove tumors with bilateral disease in 2 stages.

Two-staged pulsed photoangiolytic laser treatment by surgeons using nonionizing radiation retains elements of current phonomicrosurgery and radiotherapy models synthesizing key assets of both and comprises a significant revision of the typical surgical paradigm, which implies effective management as a solitary intervention. This is in contradistinction to radiotherapy and chemotherapy, which are incremental. For the promise of enhanced function, these nonsurgical cancer treatments have achieved acceptability despite the fact that patients have intercurrent disease during months of treatment. Moreover, it has been commonplace for decades for patients with advanced primary disease and regional metastasis to undergo incremental chemotherapy and radiotherapy (XRT) while intercurrent disease is left for 3 to 6 months. Considering this, and the fact that from microlaryngoscopic biopsy to completion of XRT is typically at least 2 months for early glottic cancer, there is no reason to believe that incremental staged endoscopic surgical treatment over the same time period will result in added risk to patients.

Salvage Endoscopic Angiolytic Potassium Titanyl Phosphate Laser Treatment of Early Glottic Cancer

Management of early glottic cancer subsequent to failed radiotherapy is challenging, especially balancing oncologic control and function preservation. Patients have frequently been incentivized against surgical management, which is why radiotherapy was selected as initial treatment. This orientation compounds the difficulty in discussions about surgical management after recurrence. Typically, endoscopic salvage is less morbid than transcervical partial laryngectomy and clearly desirable over total laryngectomy. However, there are appropriate concerns about the efficacy of endoscopic salvage and the overarching impact on larynx preservation and survival.

Given the success with endoscopic angiolytic KTP laser treatment of previously nonradiated T1 and T2 glottic cancer, the author examined previous results treating similar-sized lesions after failed radiotherapy.[19] This investigation reported on the first 20 patients who failed radiation therapy elsewhere for early glottic cancer and were treated by endoscopic angiolytic KTP laser treatment.

The presentation of the geographic tumor recurrence in the 20 patients revealed T1aN0M0-4, T1bN0M0-1, T2aN0M0-1, and T2bN0M0-14. After KTP laser salvage treatment, 4 of 20 patients (20%) developed local recurrence (all bilateral T2) and required subsequent total laryngectomy; 3 of 20 patients (15%) ultimately died of disease. The remaining 16 patients (80%) were free of disease at least 2 years subsequent to endoscopic salvage, with an average follow-up of 39 months.

This investigation provided preliminary evidence that angiolytic KTP laser salvage treatment of early glottic cancer is an effective treatment after failed radiation. Larger cohorts and longer follow-up are necessary to establish incontrovertible efficacy.

ADVANCED GLOTTIC CANCER
Extended Open Partial Laryngectomy with Aortic Homograft Reconstruction

Classical extended partial laryngectomy methods are often constrained by the balance of achieving an adequate oncological resection with retaining enough structural cartilaginous scaffolding and internal soft tissues to achieve tracheotomy decannulation. Local soft tissues and/or regional flaps typically close the defect adequately but also collapse and narrow the intralaryngeal airway lumen, frequently limiting the ability to decannulate the patient.

In addition, wide-field transcervical partial laryngectomy (TPL) is done infrequently today due to the popularity of chemotherapy–radiotherapy treatment regimens and limited enthusiasm for TPL after failed radiotherapy. Consequently, the author sought to identify a new reconstructive technique that would provide an alternative to total laryngectomy in as many patients as possible. In 2009, they initiated wide-field reconstruction of extended partial laryngectomy defects with cryopreserved homograft aorta **(Fig. 5)**.

Although the author has done over 40 procedures, of which greater than 10 were done for laryngotracheal airway stenosis, the initial pilot investigation was published in 2012.[20] In this study, 15 patients underwent single-stage wide-field TPL with cryopreserved aortic homograft reconstruction; 8 of 15 patient had failed prior radiotherapy. At least 40% of the cricoid circumference was resected in 8 of 15 patients. All 15 patients had their tracheotomy tube decannulated and had laryngeal phonation, while 14 of 15 patients resumed oral intake. There were no major surgical complications. It was common to endoscopically debride portions of the aortic graft that did not integrate in postradiation cases, but this did not lead to a laryngocutaneous fistula

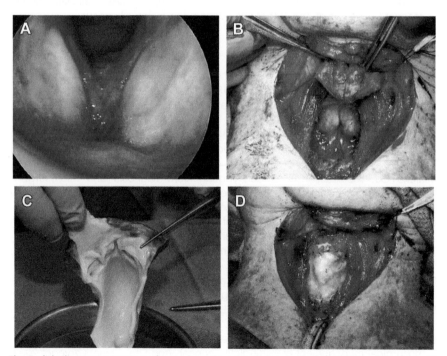

Fig. 5. (*A*) Clinic examination of a medium–large recurrence of a left glottic carcinoma with substantial extension to the subglottis and contralateral right vocal fold. (*B*) The specimen is shown including the glottis and subglottis. The undersurface of the false cords is seen remaining in the patient. (*C*) The arch of the aortic homograft will be used for the reconstruction. (*D*) The aortic homograft is sutured in position to replace the resected areas of the cartilage framework.

or prevent decannulation. Cryopreserved aortic homograft is a new, reliable, and versatile reconstructive option for performing conservation laryngeal cancer surgery that allows for airway, swallowing, and voice preservation. It is remarkable that there had been prior bench work using aortic homograft for tracheal reconstruction over 50 years ago[21] and renewed interest in recent years.[22]

Reliably replacing the aforementioned volume of laryngeal cartilage framework with consistent restoration of airway and swallowing function had not been achieved previously. The cryopreserved aortic homograft is unique in several aspects. It is essentially an acellular scaffold, so that chemical immunotherapy is unnecessary. The aortic homograft is pliant and retains its rheology in a tubular form, which maintains the airway lumen. The graft is texturally robust so that it is easy to suture into place as a patch, and its use requires routine surgical oncologic skills.

The aortic homograft appears to be extremely tolerant of exposure to upper aerodigestive tract refluxate and microbial flora, while maintaining its structural integrity following implantation despite the barotrauma associated with coughing. Based on the author's observations, there is ingrowth of microcirculation from the soft tissues of the neck, which maintains the viability of the graft. However, there is a prolonged period of intralumenal granulation in the airway (2–4 months) prior to epithelialization that is similar to wide-field endoscopic resections. This is more substantial in previously irradiated patients but does not preclude decannulation during this period. In the future, it is likely that these grafts will be seeded with patients' mucosal epithelium retrieved in a clinic biopsy, prior to the cancer resection, to hasten epithelialization of the reconstruction, which the author has observed to eventually occur.

REFERENCES

1. Fraenkel B. First healing of a laryngeal cancer taken out through the natural passages. Archiv fur Klinische Chirurgie 1886;12:281–6.
2. Lynch RC. Suspension laryngoscopy and its accomplishments. Ann Otol Rhinol Laryngol 1915;24:429–46.
3. Lynch RC. Intrinsic carcinoma of the larynx, with a second report of the cases operated on by suspension and dissection. Trans Am Laryngol Assoc 1920;40: 119–26.
4. Jako GJ, Kleinsasser O. Endolaryngeal micro-diagnosis and microsurgery. Reprint from the Annual Meeting of the American Medical Association. 1966.
5. Jako GJ. Laser surgery of the vocal cords. Laryngoscope 1972;82:2204–15.
6. Strong MS, Jako GJ. Laser surgery of the larynx: early clinical experience with continuous CO2 laser. Ann Otol Rhinol Laryngol 1972;81:791–8.
7. Strong MS. Laser excision of carcinoma of the larynx. Laryngoscope 1975;85: 1286–9.
8. Vaughan CW. Transoral laryngeal surgery using the CO2 laser. Laboratory experiments and clinical experience. Laryngoscope 1978;88:1399–420.
9. Vaughan CW, Strong MS, Jako GJ. Laryngeal carcinoma: transoral treatment using the CO2 laser. Am J Surg 1978;136:490–3.
10. Zeitels SM, Hillman RE, Franco RA, et al. Voice and treatment outcome from phonosurgical management of early glottic cancer. Ann Otol Rhinol Laryngol 2002; 111(Suppl 190):1–20.
11. Zeitels SM, Jarboe J, Franco RA. Phonosurgical reconstruction of early glottic cancer. Laryngoscope 2001;111:1862–5.
12. Zeitels SM. Optimizing voice after endoscopic partial laryngectomy. Otolaryngol Clin North Am 2004;37(3):627–36.

13. Zeitels SM, Burns JA, Hillman RH, et al. Photoangiolytic laser treatment of early glottic cancer: a new management strategy. Ann Otol Rhinol Laryngol 2008; 117(Suppl 199):1–24.

14. Folkman J. Clinical applications of research on angiogenesis. N Engl J Med 1995; 333:1757–63.

15. Zeitels SM. Atlas of phonomicrosurgery and other endolaryngeal procedures for benign and malignant disease. San Diego (CA): Singular; 2001.

16. Zeitels SM, Akst L, Burns JA, et al. Office based 532nm pulsed-KTP laser treatment of glottal papillomatosis and dysplasia. Ann Otol Rhinol Laryngol 2006;115: 679–85.

17. Zeitels SM, Burns JA. Oncologic efficacy of angiolytic KTP laser treatment of early glottic cancer. Ann Otol Rhinol Laryngol 2014;123:840–6.

18. Friedman AM, Hillman RE, Landau-Zemer T, et al. Voice outcomes for photoangiolytic ktp laser treatment of early glottic cancer. Ann Otol Rhinol Laryngol 2013;122(3):151–8.

19. Barbu A, Burns JA, Lopez-Guerra G, et al. Salvage endoscopic angiolytic KTP laser treatment of early glottic cancer after failed radiotherapy. Ann Otol Rhinol Laryngol 2013;122:235–9.

20. Zeitels SMW, Wain JC, Barbu AM, et al. Aortic homograft reconstruction of partial laryngectomy defects: a new technique. Ann Otol Rhinol Laryngol 2012;121: 301–6.

21. Pressman JJ, Simon MB. Observations upon the experimental repair of the trachea using autogenous aorta and polyethylene tubes. Surg Gynecol Obstet 1958;106(1):56–62.

22. Martinod E, Seguin A, Pfeuty K, et al. Long-term evaluation of the replacement of the trachea with an autologous aortic graft. Ann Thorac Surg 2003;75(5):1572–8 [discussion: 1578].

Voice Restoration After Total Laryngectomy

Christopher G. Tang, MD[a], Catherine F. Sinclair, MD[b],*

KEYWORDS

- Total laryngectomy • Voice restoration • Electrolarynx • Esophageal speech
- Tracheoesophageal puncture

KEY POINTS

- Loss of voice after total laryngectomy can lead to a significant decrease in a patient's quality of life, which can be improved with voice restoration.
- The 3 main modalities of voice restoration are esophageal speech, electrolarynx, and tracheoesophageal puncture.
- Esophageal speech is the most difficult to teach and for patients to learn; however, it is the most economical.
- Speech with the electrolarynx is easier to learn than esophageal speech, but requires the purchase and maintenance of an electrolarynx device.
- Tracheoesophageal puncture with voice prosthesis placement is the gold standard for voice restoration and can be done at the time of total laryngectomy or as a secondary procedure afterward.

HISTORY OF VOICE RESTORATION

Achieving voice in the absence of a functional larynx has been described for more than 150 years.[1] In 1859, Czermak and colleagues[1,2] described a girl with laryngeal stenosis who achieved voice by deflecting airflow from a tracheostomy to the tongue base. In 1874 at the third Congress of the German Company of Surgeons in Berlin, the first case of creating intelligible speech after total laryngectomy (TL) was described by Gussenbauer[3] when he fitted Billroth's first TL patient with a reedlike device mounted onto a double-lumen tracheostomy tube with a port extending into the pharynx. Since then numerous surgical modifications and devices have been described, including

Disclosures: The authors have no financial disclosures.
[a] New York Center for Voice and Swallowing Disorders, 425 West 59th Street, 10th Floor, New York, NY 10019, USA; [b] Department of Otolaryngology, Mount Sinai Icahn School of Medicine, 425 West 59th Street, 10th Floor, New York, NY 10019, USA
* Corresponding author.
E-mail address: casinclair@chpnet.org

esophageal speech in the mid-nineteenth century, electrical devices for sound generation in the early nineteenth century, and then creation of mucosal or skin fistulas directing air from the lungs to the upper esophagus and pharynx and implantation of unidirectional prosthetic valves between the trachea and upper esophagus in the mid-twentieth century.[1]

OVERVIEW OF VOICE RESTORATION

What is voice restoration? According to the Merriam-Webster dictionary, human voice is defined as sound produced by means of the lungs and larynx or the faculty of utterance.[4] Three elements are necessary for voice production with an anatomically normal vocal tract (**Fig. 1**):

1. An air generator: during expiration, the lungs generate a burst of air, which is channeled though the larynx

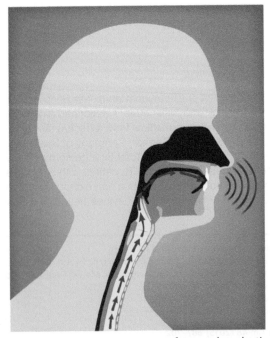

Fig. 1. Normal anatomy. Three elements are necessary for sound production: an air generator, a vibrating apparatus, and an articulating tract. (*Courtesy of* Jason Gilde, MD, Oakland, CA.)

2. A vibrating apparatus: vibrations produced by vocal fold adduction allow sound production to occur
3. An articulating tract: sound is channeled and modified through an articulating apparatus (pharynx, oral cavity) to produce an audible, understandable voice

After TL, patients maintain their air generator and articulating tract (to varying degrees depending on the extent of concomitant pharyngeal or tongue base resection). However, they lose their ability to make sound[5] (**Fig. 2**). The goal of voice restoration is to artificially create a sound source and, more specifically, to create vibratory motion of air that can be projected through and modified by the vocal tract. The 3 primary modalities of voice restoration are esophageal speech, the electrolarynx, and tracheoesophageal puncture (TEP).[6]

IMPORTANCE OF VOICE RESTORATION AFTER TOTAL LARYNGECTOMY

Numerous studies have shown that psychosocial quality of life (QOL) decreases dramatically after TL. A study of 150 patients by Babin and colleagues[7] suggests that there are significant increases in feelings of solitude after TL and that voice deprivation is a limiting factor in social relationships, tending to push individuals into social withdrawal. Reduced sexual enjoyment and libido are also common problems after laryngeal and hypopharyngeal cancer surgery.[8] Thus, successful treatment of laryngeal cancer cannot be measured by survival rates alone.

Rapid, effective restoration of voice and speech is one of the primary focuses of postoperative TL rehabilitation and is pivotal to the prevention of potential psychosocial and economic consequences.[9] One study showed that indwelling vocal

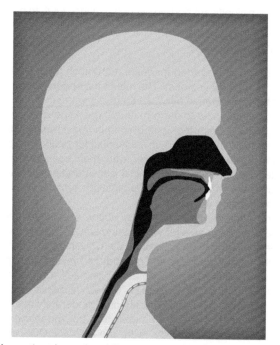

Fig. 2. After TL the patient loses the ability to make sound. (*Courtesy of* Jason Gilde, MD, Oakland, CA.)

prostheses improved QOL, self-esteem, and sexual function ($P<.05$) via several validated tests, including the World Health Organization Quality of Life–BREF, Beck Depression Inventory, Rosenberg Self-Esteem Scale, and the Arizona Sexual Experience Scale.[10] In another study on 113 patients in a developing world community, QOL scores on the European Organisation for Research and Treatment of Cancer QOL Questionnaire were significantly higher in those patients with voice restoration after TL compared with those without voice restoration.[11] Some studies also suggest that posttreatment QOL in patients who have undergone TL with vocal rehabilitation is comparable with that of patients who have undergone laryngeal preservation (chemo) radiation therapies. A study by Finizia and Bergman[12] suggests that successful speech rehabilitation with a TEP after laryngectomy may be as effective as conservative treatment with radiotherapy for laryngeal cancer with regard to psychosocial adjustment and functional ability, as measured with generic QOL instruments. In a study by Schuster and colleagues[13] that evaluated TL patients with TEP voice restoration, patients' social functioning, vitality, and mental health were not excessively limited; overall mental health and vitality were significantly better than for patients with other chronic diseases, such as heart or renal failure or hepatitis C, and general health was similar to that of a standard population. Another study by Eadie and colleagues[14] suggests that patients had a high level of self-perceived QOL after TEP in the domains of communication, eating, pain, and emotion that was empirically better than results found in a previous study involving individuals who had undergone TL without voice restoration. Possible reasons cited for the improved self-reported QOL among patients having voice restoration included use of tracheoesophageal speech for postlaryngectomy communication, a higher level of education, and membership in a support group.

Overall, the ability to communicate and converse with others is essential to an individual's QOL and spans the gambit of people's activities of daily living. Voice restoration after TL enables a significant portion of such patients' QOL to be returned to them.

PATIENT EVALUATION OVERVIEW

All patients who are to be evaluated for voice restoration after TL should have a preoperative speech therapy assessment. The role of the speech therapist is pivotal in all 3 modalities of voice rehabilitation because there is a learning curve for all techniques. Patients need to be taught how to perform esophageal speech, use an electrolarynx, or use their TEP, and a speech therapist trained in vocal rehabilitative techniques is best equipped to provide that training. It is essential for patients to plan for a specific voice rehabilitation method preoperatively with their speech therapists and then implement that technique after TL. Financial considerations should also be taken into account because the different vocal rehabilitation methods all have variable costs, especially in the developing world.[15]

Preoperative and postoperative vocal dysfunction should be longitudinally documented using one or more of several voice rating scales. Popular scales include the Voice Handicap Index 10 (VHI-10) as well as the University of Washington Quality of Life scale (UWQOL). A study by Eadie and colleagues[16] investigated potential relationships between speech intelligibility, acceptability, and self-reported QOL after TL and compared the UWQOL and VHI-10 scales. Speech acceptability and intelligibility varied across the samples, with acceptability only moderately related to intelligibility ($r = 0.41$; $P<.05$). The only statistically significant, but moderate, relationship was found between speech acceptability with the UWQOLQOL speech subscore ($r = 0.46$; $P<.05$) suggesting that it may be a more appropriate rating scale for voice assessment after TL than the VHI-10.

ESOPHAGEAL SPEECH
Overview

Esophageal speech is produced by insufflation of air into the esophagus, essentially by swallowing air. The air is then released in a controlled manner back through the esophagus allowing the mucosa of the upper esophagus/neopharynx to vibrate. Using the vibrations of the pharyngeal/esophageal mucosa as a sound source, the vibratory air column is channeled through the articulatory apparatus of the upper pharynx and oral cavity, where it can be modified and modulated to produce understandable voice (**Fig. 3**).

Patient Evaluation

According to several studies, esophageal speech is more difficult than other methods to learn to use. However, advantages compared with other voice rehabilitation methods include low cost (no need to purchase an external vibratory device such as a tracheal-esophageal prosthesis or an electrolarynx) and no need for additional surgeries. All TL patients who have access to a professional trained in teaching esophageal speech would qualify for this technique, although patients with tight cricopharyngeal musculature or who develop esophageal or pharyngeal stenoses postoperatively have difficulty with voice production by this method. This technique is used most commonly in developing countries secondary to its low cost.[15,17]

Management Goals

The main goal for esophageal speech is to restore voice with minimal surgical intervention. For patients who do not wish further surgery or the possible complications

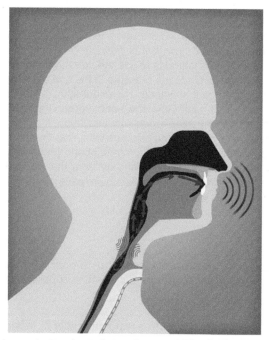

Fig. 3. Esophageal speech. Esophageal speech is produced by insufflation of air into the esophagus, essentially by swallowing air. The air is then released in a controlled manner back through the esophagus allowing the mucosa of the upper esophagus/neopharynx to vibrate. (*Courtesy of* Jason Gilde, MD, Oakland, CA.)

associated with a TEP, esophageal speech may be a viable alternative. In addition, as stated previously, no external devices need to be purchased or maintained. As stated by Staffieri and colleagues,[15] there is a steep learning curve and many patients find it difficult to learn initially, but it remains the most economical option of all voice restoration techniques.

There are many difficulties in learning esophageal speech. In addition to patient difficulty in learning how to perform esophageal speech, there are often obstacles for primary speech therapists in teaching esophageal speech. Most speech therapists do not use esophageal speech as their primary communication modality because they all have larynges. Because they have not had TL, any attempt at showing esophageal speech by the speech therapist allows the swallowed air to pass through the laryngeal apparatus, making it innately different than for someone who has had a TL.

Because surgery is not performed, there are no surgical complications. The main nonsurgical complications are failure to learn how to perform esophageal speech and potential loss of voice should esophageal or pharyngeal stenosis or significant cricopharyngeal muscle spasms evolve. Cricopharyngeal spasm can be managed conservatively with exercises supervised by a speech therapist (in mild to moderate cases) or, if this fails, chemically with botulinum toxin–induced muscle paralysis or surgically by division of the cricopharyngeus muscle. Division of the cricopharyngeus muscle at the time of TL is advisable if esophageal speech is to be considered and care must be taken to divide all visible muscle fibers. Effects of botulinum toxin for cricopharyngeal spasm last approximately 4 to 6 months before the patient needs to be reinjected. Surgical cricopharyngeal muscle division is associated with risks of bleeding, perforation, and recurrence from inadequate muscle division.

Treatment

Esophageal speech can be performed through 2 techniques, both based on the principle of pressure gradients and how matter flows from areas of higher pressure to areas of lower pressure. One method is to use the oral cavity/lip muscles to increase air pressure in the oral cavity. Once the pressure in the oral cavity is greater than that exerted by the cricopharyngeal sphincter, the esophagus is insufflated as air flows from the high-pressure oral cavity into the esophagus. The second method is by decreasing the pressure in the esophagus with inhalation. If a rapid breath is taken, the thorax expands rapidly, allowing the pressure within the thoracic cavity, and hence the esophagus, to decrease dramatically. Atmospheric pressure would be greater than the pressure in the esophagus, allowing air from the atmosphere to enter the esophagus via the vocal tract. Both methods require extensive training and perseverance with speech therapy is essential.[18]

ELECTROLARYNX
Overview

Voice restoration with an electrolarynx occurs by producing vibrations in the oral cavity or pharyngeal mucosa with an external vibrating apparatus (**Fig. 4**).

Patient Evaluation

Benefits of using the electrolarynx for voice restoration after TL include lack of need for further surgical procedures (compared with TEP) and ease of learning (compared with esophageal speech). Disadvantages include the mechanical sound of the voice produced, which, as shown in several studies, causes much greater patient-perceived vocal handicap compared with TEP voice.[19,20] Patients need to purchase and

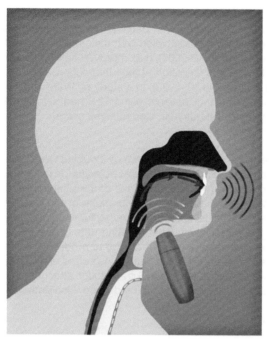

Fig. 4. Electrolarynx. Voice restoration with an electrolarynx occurs by producing vibrations in the oral cavity or pharyngeal mucosa with an external vibrating apparatus. (*Courtesy of Jason Gilde, MD, Oakland, CA.*)

maintain an electrolarynx device, and, in low-income populations and developing countries, the device is often outside the economic range.[15,17] Classically the electrolarynx has been a hand-held device and thus manual dexterity can be an issue. However, a recently developed device that uses an electromyography (EMG) transducer attached to the strap muscles to activate a vibratory source allows hands-free vocalization.[21] The electrolarynx is reliant on the articulatory musculature, and thus loss of articulatory musculature during surgical resection can have consequences for intelligible electrolarynx use.

Management Goals

The primary management goal is to achieve understandable voice by use of the patient's own articulatory apparatus with minimal intervention. For patients who do not wish further surgery or the possible complications associated with a TEP, and patients who either cannot vocalize with esophageal speech or choose not to, the electrolarynx may be a viable restorative option.

Several studies have shown that voice with the electrolarynx, although superior to esophageal speech, is still worse in quality than voice restoration with a TEP. In a study by Finizia and Bergman,[12] patients who had voice restoration with an electrolarynx displayed worse Sickness Impact Profile (SIP) and Hospital Anxiety and Depression Scale scores compared with TL patients with a TEP and with patients with laryngeal cancer who had laryngeal preservation with primary radiation therapy. In 10 of 12 SIP categories, the numerically highest proportion of patients with clinically important dysfunction (SIP scores >10) was found in the electrolarynx group.[12] Another study by

Clements and colleagues[20] shows the superior quality of voice with TEPs compared with the electrolarynx. Compared with patients using the electrolarynx, TL patients with TEP were significantly more satisfied with their speech ($P<.001$), perceived their speech to be of better quality ($P<.001$), had improved ability to communicate over the telephone ($P<.001$), had less limitation of their interactions with others ($P<.004$), and rated their overall QOL higher ($P = .23$). In a study by Ward and colleagues,[22] statistical comparison revealed that patients using TEP had significantly lower levels of disability, handicap, and distress than electrolarynx users.

Treatment

As stated previously, the electrolarynx works by inducing vibrations of oral or pharyngeal mucosa by an external device. The electrolarynx device can be placed on the neck externally and causes indirect vibrations of the pharyngeal mucosa, or can be placed intraorally, thereby causing direct vibrations of the oral cavity mucosa. The intraoral technique involves using a small vibrating tube that is inserted into the mouth and placed deep in the oral cavity. This vibrating tube is then laid against the buccal mucosa, pharyngeal mucosa, or base of tongue to produce the vibration, depending on the technique and preference of the patient. As stated previously, there has been a new device developed that uses an EMG transducer attached to the strap muscles that activates a vibratory source to allow hands-free vocalization.[21]

TRACHEOESOPHAGEAL PUNCTURE
Overview

TEP is the gold standard for voice rehabilitation after TL. A TEP allows a patient to channel air from the lungs through a puncture site in the back wall of the trachea, into the esophagus, and up through the pharynx and mouth. This technique allows air pressure generated from the lungs to go through the esophagus where the esophageal mucosa acts as a vibrating apparatus and into the oral cavity where it can be modulated by articulatory mechanisms (**Fig. 5**).

Patient Evaluation

Several studies have shown that voice restoration with TEP is superior to both the electrolarynx and esophageal speech in that it is technically easier to learn to use and vocal quality is superior.[12,20,22] Access to a speech therapist in the preoperative, perioperative, and postoperative settings is essential for proper TEP management, including learning to use the TEP, care for the puncture site, and replacement of the prosthesis with device malfunctions. A potential disadvantage of TEP is the expense of the prostheses, which can be prohibitive for low-income patients and those in the developing world.[15] The speech prosthesis can be placed primarily at the time of TL or secondarily at a second surgery, typically some weeks after TL. Several factors are important in determining the timing of valve placement and these are discussed later.

Management Goals

As stated earlier, several studies have shown that voice restoration with TEP is superior to both the electrolarynx and esophageal speech. Criteria for TEP include favorable anatomy, ability to cover the stoma, and stoma size. Patients need to have favorable anatomy for placement of a TEP because nonanatomic positioning of the final stoma can make prosthesis placement and use difficult. In addition, patients need to have the ability to cover the stoma physically, and patients who have had strokes, musculoskeletal disorders, or amputations may have difficulty manipulating and covering the stoma. Free-flap pharyngeal reconstruction is not a contraindication to TEP placement.[23]

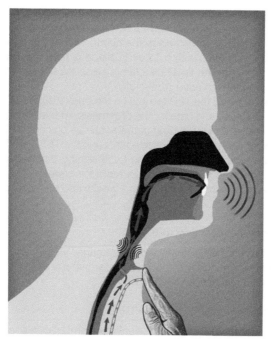

Fig. 5. A TEP allows a patient to channel air from the lungs through a puncture site in the back wall of the trachea, into the esophagus, and up through the pharynx mouth. (*Courtesy of* Jason Gilde, MD, Oakland, CA.)

Preoperative Planning and Preparation

There are several patient and disease factors that should be considered when determining whether a patient should have a primary or secondary TEP. In the past, TEP was most commonly performed secondarily because of concerns about increased complications with primary TEP. Pharyngocutaneous fistula (PCF) rates after salvage TL approach 33% and thus many surgeons opted to perform secondary TEPs in this patient population.[24–26] Development of PCF after salvage TL can be minimized by the use of vascularized free-tissue reconstruction.[27] Several recent studies have found that there is no increased rate of complications with primary TEP placement and that there is no difference in complication rates of patients who have primary versus secondary TEP.[28–30] A study by Sinclair and colleagues[23] showed that the presence of a microvascular free flap is not a contraindication to placement of a TEP and there was no difference in the early complication rate for primary versus secondary TEP following TL with concurrent free-flap reconstruction. Moreover, a similar number of patients who had TL with free-flap reconstructions achieved intelligible speech with either primary or secondary TEP placement. Performance of secondary TEP may also be preferred in certain cases for reasons including timing of adjuvant therapies, traveling constraints, and medical comorbidities.[23]

PERIOPERATIVE CONSIDERATIONS
Primary Tracheoesophageal Puncture

Primary TEP is performed at the time of TL. After the TL is performed, the cricopharyngeus muscle is divided. In order to determine optimal TEP placement, it is helpful to construct the inferior part of the stoma by suturing the inferior aspect of the trachea to skin. A hemostatic clamp is then inserted into the esophageal lumen under direct vision and anterior pressure is applied to the clamp to that that the posterior wall of the trachea tents up. A scalpel with a 15 or 11 blade is then used to cut through the posterior tracheal wall onto the tip of the clamp. Because the esophagus is exposed during TL, there is no need to enter transorally.

It is important to not place the TEP too low on the back wall of the stoma because it may be more difficult to use and care for the prosthesis. At this time a vocal prosthesis can be inserted primarily, or a red rubber catheter can be placed to allow for a fistula to form.[31] A red rubber catheter is then inserted through the TEP and directed down the neopharynx into the esophagus so that the tip is resting distally. A cricopharyngeal myotomy can be performed at this time to facilitate speech. The catheter is then secured. The catheter is normally changed in 2 weeks and the vocal prosthesis placed at that time.[32]

Secondary Tracheoesophageal Puncture

Secondary placement of TEP can be performed either in the clinic or under general anesthesia. Although traditionally performed under general anesthesia, placement of TEP in the clinic is a novel and efficient method.

Secondary Tracheoesophageal Puncture in Clinic

Placement of a secondary TEP in clinic is usually performed with a modified Seldinger/ reverse puncture technique. As a highly effective and cost-saving procedure, this can be performed in most centers. The first series of secondary TEP performed under local anesthesia was published by Desyatnikova and colleagues[33] in 2001. This technique involved inserting a nasopharyngoscope transnasally with visualization of the hypopharynx while the procedure was performed. However, visualization of the esophagus was not performed with this technique. The technique of secondary TEP performed via transnasal esophagoscopy, as described by Bach and colleagues,[34] is discussed later. Several additional modifications have been described in the literature.[35,36]

Procedural Approach

With the patient sitting upright, the nasal cavity and oral cavity are anesthetized with topical anesthetic. Lidocaine with epinephrine is infiltrated through the stoma into the posterior tracheal wall at the site of the proposed TEP site. A transnasal esophagoscope is inserted through the nose, nasopharynx, and neopharynx into the esophagus. Areas of stenosis may need to be dilated before insertion. Identification of the TEP site can be made from within the esophageal lumen by pressing externally at the posterior tracheal wall with an instrument such as a hemostat or a bayonet forceps. The TEP site can also be visualized externally by the light at the end of the esophagoscope against the posterior tracheal wall. Once this is confirmed, an 18-gauge needle is inserted through the posterior tracheal wall. Care is taken so that the needle can be seen entering the esophageal lumen under direct visualization from the esophagoscope. A scalpel blade can be used to cut on the needle, or the needle can be removed and a scalpel used to make a stab incision at the site of the needle. A hemostat is inserted to enlarge the opening. Air insufflation of the esophagus can assist with this part of the procedure and careful observation through the esophagoscope ensures that there is no contact with the posterior esophageal wall. TEP dilators are then passed through the puncture site and an appropriately sized voice prosthesis is inserted via a gel capsule technique.[34]

SECONDARY TRACHEOESOPHAGEAL PUNCTURE IN THE OPERATING ROOM
Patient Positioning

The procedure is performed under general anesthesia with the patient positioned supine. After general anesthesia is induced, an endotracheal tube is placed into the tracheal stoma to ventilate the patient. This tube can be removed intermittently so the surgeon can work on the tracheoesophageal wall.

Procedural Approach

The TEP was first described in the 1970s[37] and improved on by Singer and Blom[38] in the 1980s.[38–40] Although there are many variations of the original surgery, the basic steps for the TEP are described here.

A cervical esophagoscope is inserted transorally into the neopharynx and down the esophagus with the bevel facing anteriorly (**Fig. 6**). The esophagoscope is advanced until it can be palpated through the laryngeal stoma. An 18-gauge needle is inserted through the back wall of the tracheostoma and into the lumen of the esophagoscope under direct visualization through the esophagoscope (**Fig. 7**). At this time, the opening can be enlarged using sharp dissection and a voice prosthesis placed immediately, or a red rubber catheter placed to allow better epithelialization of the fistula.

If the surgeon decides to place a red rubber catheter to allow epithelialization, a 24-gauge guidewire can be passed through the needle into the esophagoscope (**Fig. 8**). Endoscopic esophageal forceps are used to grasp the wire through the esophagoscope and pulled through the esophagoscope. The tracheoesophageal opening is widened around the guidewire with a scalpel and hemostat. The guidewire

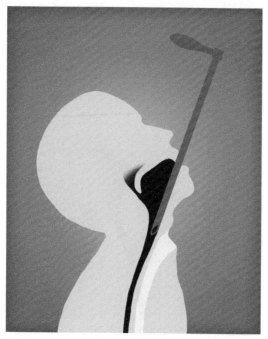

Fig. 6. Secondary TEP: step 1. A cervical esophagoscope is inserted transorally into the neopharynx and down the esophagus with the bevel facing anteriorly. (*Courtesy of* Jason Gilde, MD, Oakland, CA.)

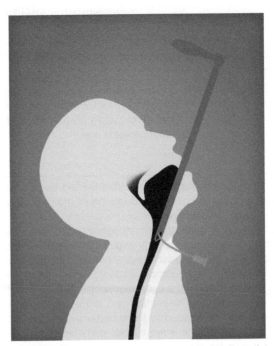

Fig. 7. Secondary TEP: step 2. The esophagoscope is advanced until it can be palpated through the laryngeal stoma. An 18-gauge needle is inserted through the back wall of the tracheostoma and into the lumen of the esophagoscope under direct visualization. (*Courtesy of* Jason Gilde, MD, Oakland, CA.)

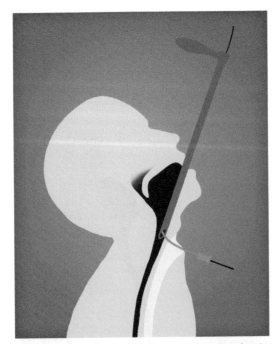

Fig. 8. Secondary TEP: step 3. If a voice prosthesis is not placed at the time of TEP, a red rubber catheter can be placed to allow for fistula formation. A 24-gauge guidewire is then passed through the needle into the esophagoscope and the red rubber catheter is attached to the needle. (*Courtesy of* Jason Gilde, MD, Oakland, CA.)

is then tied to a red rubber catheter, and the guidewire removed transorally from the esophagoscope. The proximal end of the red rubber catheter is sutured next to the tracheostoma. The distal end (within the esophagoscope) is then grasped with alligator forceps and advanced distally into the distal esophagus where it rests. Again, after 2 weeks, the red rubber catheter is removed and replaced with a voice prosthesis.[32]

Potential Complications and Management

Perioperative complications include breaking of the guidewire, esophageal laceration, and perforation. To avoid these complications, ensure that the fistula is large enough to avoid pressure on the catheter and ensure that there is no free edge on the guidewire. Patients with chronic medical issues that cause delayed wound healing (eg, diabetes, recent neck irradiation, malnutrition) may have delayed healing of the TEP site and it is advisable to optimize management of underlying medical conditions and/or time after neck irradiation before TEP placement.

Potential postoperative complications include valve displacement, stomal stenosis, and TEP blockage from debris or secretions. Inappropriately placed TEPs may predispose the patient to many complications. A TEP placed too inferiorly could be difficult to change. Moreover, inappropriate placement of the TEP can make it difficult to cover the stoma without covering the TEP. Stenosis of the tracheostoma can be prevented with careful surgical technique, and can be treated by stomal dilations. TEP blockages can be alleviated by changing the vocal prosthesis. Sometimes the TEP is too large for the prosthesis, or enlarges over time. The TEP may then need to be revised surgically.[32]

Postprocedural Care

If a red rubber catheter was placed to allow epithelialization of the tracheoesophageal fistula, the red rubber catheter is removed after 10 to 14 days. Once that is removed, frequent stomal and TEP cleaning is necessary to prevent obstruction or infection. Speech therapy is essential to teach the patient how to care for the TEP/prosthesis and how to use it to vocalize.

Rehabilitation and Recovery

Patients recover quickly after TEP placements. As stated earlier, it is necessary to keep the area clean and to have follow-up with speech therapy.

OUTCOMES/COMPLICATIONS

With the Provox vocal prosthesis, one study quoted that 78% of patients rated their long-term tracheoesophageal speech as good or average. The main causes for valve replacement were obstruction, leakage, or inadequate size of the prosthesis, and granulation or leakage around the fistula.[41] In another study of 318 patients by Op de Coul and colleagues,[42] the main indications for replacement were device related, such as leakage through the prosthesis (73%) and obstruction (4%), or fistula-related, such as leakage around the prosthesis (13%), and hypertrophy and/or infection of the fistula (7%). Adverse events occurred in 11% of all replacements in one-third of the patients, and were mostly solvable by a shrinkage period, or adequate sizing and/or antibiotic treatment. Definitive closure of the tracheoesophageal fistula tract occurred in 5% of the patients. Significant clinical factors for increased device lifetime were the absence of radiotherapy ($P = .03$), and age older than 70 years ($P<.02$). The success rate with respect to voice quality (ie, fair to excellent rating) was 88%, which was significantly influenced by the extent of surgery (P<.001).[42] A study by Chone and colleagues[43] suggested that the use of radiation therapy (XRT) and patient age did not influence the success of vocal prostheses among primary and secondary TEP, with an overall success rate of 94%. With regard to TL patients in South Africa using the Provox voice prosthesis, the mean device life was 303 days and adverse events occurred in 16 patients.[44] In a study by Aust and colleagues,[45] reasons for failure included infection, radiation fibrosis, manual incoordination, cerebrovascular accident, and combination of TL and total glossectomy. The most common complication (in 2 patients) was retraction of the prosthesis into the esophagus, which was successfully managed by replacement with a longer device. In a study by Van den Hoogen and colleagues[46] comparing the Groningen, Nijdam, and Provox voice prostheses, voice rehabilitation was successful in 94% to 100% of patients 10 months after surgery. No significant overall differences were found between the 3 prostheses. No differences between the 3 prostheses were found with regard to improving voice quality over time.[46]

SUMMARY

The 3 main modalities of voice restoration after TL are esophageal speech, the electrolarynx, and a TEP. Of these, esophageal speech is the least expensive, but the most difficult to learn with the lowest quality of voice. The gold standard for voice restoration after TL is the TEP, which can be placed at the time of TL (primary), or at a later time (secondary).

REFERENCES

1. Bień S, Rinaldo A, Silver CE, et al. History of voice rehabilitation following laryngectomy. Laryngoscope 2008;118(3):453–8.
2. Weir N. Otolaryngology. An illustrated history. London: Butterworths; 1990.
3. Gussenbauer C. Ueber die erste durch Th. Billroth am Menschen ausgeführte Kehlkopf-Exstirpation und die Anwendung eines künstlichen Kehlkopfes. Arch Klin Chir Berlin 1874;17:343–56.
4. Merriam-Webster Dictionary. 2014. Available at: http://www.merriam-webster.com/dictionary/voice. Accessed October 1, 2014.
5. Elmiyeh B, Dwivedi RC, Jallali N, et al. Surgical voice restoration after total laryngectomy: an overview. Indian J Cancer 2010;47(3):239–47.
6. Perry AR, Shaw MA, Cotton S. An evaluation of functional outcomes (speech, swallowing) in patients attending speech pathology after head and neck cancer treatments(s): results and analysis at 12 months post-intervention. J Laryngol Otol 2003;117:368–81.
7. Babin E, Beynier D, Le Gall D, et al. Psychosocial quality of life in patients after total laryngectomy. Rev Laryngol Otol Rhinol (Bord) 2009;130(1):29–34.
8. Singer S, Danker H, Dietz A, et al. Sexual problems after total or partial laryngectomy. Laryngoscope 2008;118(12):2218–24.
9. Blom ED. Current status of voice restoration following total laryngectomy. Oncology (Williston Park) 2000;14(6):915–22 [discussion: 927–8, 931].
10. Polat B, Orhan KS, Kesimli MC, et al. The effects of indwelling voice prosthesis on the quality of life, depressive symptoms, and self-esteem in patients with total laryngectomy. Eur Arch Otorhinolaryngol 2014. [Epub ahead of print].
11. Varghese BT, Mathew A, Sebastian P, et al. Comparison of quality of life between voice rehabilitated and nonrehabilitated laryngectomies in a developing world community. Acta Otolaryngol 2011;131(3):310–5.

12. Finizia C, Bergman B. Health-related quality of life in patients with laryngeal cancer: a post-treatment comparison of different modes of communication. Laryngoscope 2001;111(5):918–23.
13. Schuster M, Lohscheller J, Kummer P, et al. Quality of life in laryngectomees after prosthetic voice restoration. Folia Phoniatr Logop 2003;55:211–9.
14. Eadie TL, Doyle PC. Quality of life in male TE speakers. J Rehabil Res Dev 2005; 42:115–24.
15. Staffieri A, Mostafea BE, Varghese BT, et al. Cost of tracheoesophageal prostheses in developing countries. Facing the problem from an internal perspective. Acta Otolaryngol 2006;126(1):4–9.
16. Eadie TL, Day AM, Sawin DE, et al. Auditory-perceptual speech outcomes and quality of life after total laryngectomy. Otolaryngol Head Neck Surg 2013; 148(1):82–8.
17. Xi S. Effectiveness of voice rehabilitation on vocalisation in postlaryngectomy patients: a systematic review. Int J Evid Based Healthc 2010;8(4):256–8.
18. Singer S, Wollbrück D, Dietz A, et al. Speech rehabilitation during the first year after total laryngectomy. Head Neck 2012;35:1583–90.
19. Koike M, Kobayashi N, Hirose H, et al. Speech rehabilitation after total laryngectomy. Acta Otolaryngol 2002;122(Suppl 547):107–12.
20. Clements KS, Rassekh CH, Seikaly H, et al. Communication after laryngectomy. An assessment of patient satisfaction. Arch Otolaryngol Head Neck Surg 1997; 123(5):493–6.
21. Goldstein EA, Heaton JT, Stepp CE, et al. Training effects on speech production using a hands-free electromyographically controlled electrolarynx. J Speech Lang Hear Res 2007;50(2):335–51.
22. Ward EC, Koh SK, Frisby J, et al. Differential modes of alaryngeal communication and long-term voice outcomes following pharyngolaryngectomy and laryngectomy. Folia Phoniatr Logop 2003;55(1):39–49.
23. Sinclair CF, Rosenthal EL, McColloch NL, et al. Primary versus delayed tracheoesophageal puncture for laryngopharyngectomy with free flap reconstruction. Laryngoscope 2011;121(7):1436–40.
24. Emerick KS, Tomycz L, Bradford CR, et al. Primary versus secondary tracheoesophageal puncture in salvage total laryngectomy following chemoradiation. Otolaryngol Head Neck Surg 2009;140(3):386–90.
25. Weber RS, Burkey BA, Forastiere A, et al. Outcome of salvage total laryngectomy following organ preservation therapy—the Radiation Therapy Oncology Group trial 91-11. Arch Otolaryngol Head Neck Surg 2003;129:44–9.
26. Sassler AM, Esclamado RM, Wolf GT. Surgery after organ preservation therapy—analysis of wound complications. Arch Otolaryngol Head Neck Surg 1995;121: 162–5.
27. Withrow KP, Rosenthal EL, Gourin CG, et al. Free tissue transfer to manage salvage laryngectomy defects after organ preservation failure. Laryngoscope 2007;117(5):781–4.
28. Cheng E, Ho M, Ganz C, et al. Outcomes of primary and secondary tracheoesophageal puncture: a 16-year retrospective analysis. Ear Nose Throat J 2006;85: 262–7.
29. Trudeau MD, Schuller DE, Hall DA. The timing of tracheoesophageal puncture for voice restoration: primary vs secondary. Head Neck Surg 1988;10:130–4.
30. Wenig BL, Levy J, Mullooly V, et al. Voice restoration following laryngectomy: the role of primary versus secondary tracheoesophageal puncture. Ann Otol Rhinol Laryngol 1989;98:70–3.

31. Cole I, Miller S. Total laryngectomy with primary voice restoration. Aust N Z J Surg 1992;62(4):279–82.
32. Eibling DE. Chapter 50: voice restoration after total laryngectomy. In: Meyers EN, editor. Operative otolaryngology head and neck surgery, vol. 1, 2nd edition. Philadelphia: Saunders/Elsevier; 2008. p. 431–7.
33. Desyatnikova S, Caro JJ, Andersen PE, et al. Tracheoesophageal puncture in the office setting with local anesthesia. Ann Otol Rhinol Laryngol 2001;110(7 Pt 1): 613–6.
34. Bach KK, Postma GN, Koufman JA. In-office tracheoesophageal puncture using transnasal esophagoscopy. Laryngoscope 2003;113(1):173–6.
35. Eerenstein SE, Schouwenburg PF. Secondary tracheoesophageal puncture with local anesthesia. Laryngoscope 2002;112(4):634–7.
36. Fukuhara T, Fujiwara K, Nomura K, et al. New method for in-office secondary voice prosthesis insertion under local anesthesia by reverse puncture from esophageal lumen. Ann Otol Rhinol Laryngol 2013;122(3):163–8.
37. Sisson GA, McConnel FM, Logemann JA, et al. Voice rehabilitation after laryngectomy. Results with the use of a hypopharyngeal prosthesis. Arch Otolaryngol 1975;101(3):178–81.
38. Singer MI, Blom ED. An endoscopic technique for restoration of voice after laryngectomy. Ann Otol Rhinol Laryngol 1980;89(6 Pt 1):529–33.
39. Wetmore SJ, Krueger K, Wesson K. The Singer-Blom speech rehabilitation procedure. Laryngoscope 1981;91(7):1109–17.
40. Wood BG, Rusnov MG, Tucker HM, et al. Tracheoesophageal puncture for alaryngeal voice restoration. Ann Otol Rhinol Laryngol 1981;90(5 Pt 1):492–4.
41. Makitie AA, Niemensivu R, Juvas A, et al. Postlaryngectomy voice restoration using a voice prosthesis: a single institution's ten-year experience. Ann Otol Rhinol Laryngol 2003;112:1007–10.
42. Op de Coul BMR, Hilgers FJM, Balm AJM, et al. A decade of postlaryngectomy vocal rehabilitation in 318 patients: a single institution's experience with consistent application of Provox indwelling voice prostheses. Arch Otolaryngol Head Neck Surg 2000;126:1320–8.
43. Chone CT, Spina AL, Crespo AN, et al. Speech rehabilitation after total laryngectomy: long-term results with indwelling voice prosthesis Blom-Singer. Braz J Otorhinolaryngol 2005;71:504–9.
44. Cornu AS, Vlantis AC, Elliott H, et al. Voice rehabilitation after laryngectomy with the Provox voice prosthesis in South Africa. J Laryngol Otol 2003;117:56–9.
45. Aust MR, McCaffrey TV. Early speech results with the Provox prosthesis after laryngectomy. Arch Otolaryngol Head Neck Surg 1997;123:966–8.
46. Van den Hoogen FJ, Van den Berg RJ, Oudes MJ, et al. A prospective study of speech and voice rehabilitation after total laryngectomy with the low-resistance Groningen, Nijdam and Provox voice prostheses. Clin Otolaryngol Allied Sci 1998;23(5):425–31.

Transcervical Conservation Laryngeal Surgery

An Anatomic Understanding to Enhance Functional and Oncologic Outcomes

Moustafa Mourad, MD[a], Babak Sadoughi, MD[b],*

KEYWORDS

- Transcervical conservation laryngeal surgery • Glottic carcinoma
- Supraglottic carcinoma • Open partial laryngectomy

KEY POINTS

- In order to appropriately manage and counsel patients with laryngeal cancer, the physician must not only be aware of the armamentarium of treatment options, but also have a thorough understanding of the complex laryngeal anatomy that impacts tumor growth and behavior.
- Surgical and nonsurgical approaches should be considered with appropriate referrals as indicated; surgical options include transoral and transcervical approaches.
- The fibroelastic framework of the larynx provides distinctive barriers that may limit tumor extension in the early stages, but also guide predictable migration patterns in advanced cases.
- The paraglottic spaces form a conduit for extension to different laryngeal regions, which must be understood to better determine optimal treatment options.
- Understanding the distinctive anatomic associations within the larynx will enhance tumor mapping, and allow for superior outcomes.

 Videos of Laryngeal Framework Anatomy; Horizontal Partial Laryngectomies; SGPL; SCPL-CHEP; and SCPL-CHP accompany this article at http://www.oto.theclinics.com/

BACKGROUND

The understanding of the complex 3-dimensional anatomy of the larynx presents as a challenge to many beginning surgeons and clinicians. When presented with carcinoma of the larynx, an insufficient grasp of this intricate landscape may hamper the

a Department of Otolaryngology, New York Eye and Ear Infirmary, Mount Sinai Health System, 310 East 14 Street, New York, NY 10003, USA; b Department of Otolaryngology - Head and Neck Surgery, The Sean Parker Institute for the Voice, Weill Cornell Medical College, 1305 York Avenue, 5th Floor, New York, NY 10021, USA
* Corresponding author.
E-mail address: bas9049@med.cornell.edu

Otolaryngol Clin N Am 48 (2015) 703–715
http://dx.doi.org/10.1016/j.otc.2015.04.014
0030-6665/15/$ – see front matter © 2015 Elsevier Inc. All rights reserved.

clinician's ability to adequately counsel, refer, and direct appropriate therapeutic options for the patient. The objective of this article is to enhance the reader's understanding of the critical anatomic structures that influence the evolution of laryngeal carcinoma and its functional impact on the larynx, in order to define the indications and contraindications of conservation laryngeal surgery.

Conservation options in ablative laryngeal surgery include both transoral and open transcervical approaches. The mainstay surgical treatment option for most early lesions is typically via a transoral approach, with shorter hospitalizations, lower morbidity, and improved functional results.[1] However, this review will focus on transcervical approaches and discuss their seminal anatomic principles. Open approaches can be considered in situations where exposure is inadequate for transoral resection, or the transoral technique is not in the purview of the institution, as well as for salvage surgery after radiation failure. This topic will serve as a guide for clinicians seeking to understand management options beyond transoral laser surgery, radiation therapy, and total laryngectomy.

The different categories of open organ preservation surgery and their indications and contraindications will be summarized. The anatomic bases for these indications will be subsequently described.

GUIDING PRINCIPLES AND UNDERSTANDING OF TUMOR SPREAD

One should have familiarity with the complex normal laryngeal anatomy and the ability to establish an accurate assessment of tumor extent. Tumor mapping is performed through a combination of office-based, surgical clinical examination, and radiographic studies. The clinician should be astute to the extent of mucosal involvement, depth of invasion, as well as mobility of the vocal folds and arytenoids.

The guiding principles of organ-sparing surgery are to provide oncologically sound outcomes while preserving the sphincteric, respiratory, and phonatory capabilities of the larynx. An attempt should be made to maintain the 3 fundamental functions by preserving at least 1 functional cricoarytenoid unit. In addition, the cricoid cartilage is the only complete cartilaginous ring in the airway, and must be preserved in order to prevent airway compromise.

Anatomic Point #1

Bilateral compromise of the cricoarytenoid units or the structural integrity of the cricoid cartilage should preclude organ preservation surgery as an option.

Certain properties of the laryngeal cartilaginous and fibrous framework should be taken into account, particularly in the way they impact tumor growth and extension capabilities (**Fig. 1**, Video 1). In Brennan and colleagues'[2] review of the literature, the majority of squamous cell carcinoma (78%) invasion was through direct extension, with only 10% (11 of 107) of cases exhibiting documented involvement via lymphatic spread.

Early glottic lesions may respect the fibroelastic framework of the larynx, whereas larger lesions may utilize the framework for further extension. Laryngeal regions most susceptible to spread are at the anterior angle of the thyroid cartilage and the cricothyroid membrane.[3,4] Histopathologic studies have shown that tumor spread seems to occur along collagen bundles where the connective tissue membranes attach to the cartilage. As the tumor expands, it causes expansion of the collagen bundles, resulting in a direct pathway for the spread of the lesion through the

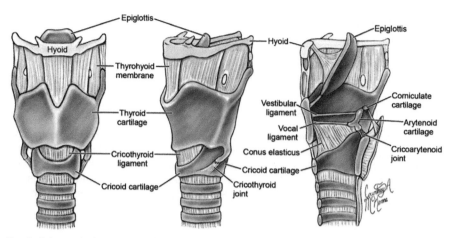

Fig. 1. Schematic description of laryngeal cartilaginous framework. The framework serves as an impedance to early glottic lesions, but may facilitate the progression of advanced lesions in a predictable pattern. (Printed with permission from © Mount Sinai Health System.)

perichondrium.[1,4] This subsequently makes the cricothyroid membrane and anterior commissure ligament more susceptible to direct extension of tumor.

Perichondrium may provide a barrier to direct extension of laryngeal tumors. However, once the tumor has compromised this barrier, it may allow for the tumor to spread in a subperichondrial plane behind an intact perichondrium. This may contribute to understaging of laryngeal cancers and inaccurate assessment of thyroid cartilage involvement.[2,5] Recognizing the latter is critical in directing appropriate management when considering open laryngeal procedures. Direct extension may occur through areas of ossification and osteoclast formation, or areas of high vascularity.[3,4,6–8] Furthermore, thyroid cartilage involvement may occur through areas devoid of perichondrium (eg, Broyles ligament insertion at the anterior commissure) along collagen bundles.[3,4]

The anterior commissure is an area of epithelial confluence of the anterior vocal folds, covering the posterior aspect of the thyroid cartilage at the midline.[9] Inserted onto the anterior commissure is Broyles ligament, which is a continuation of the vocal ligament. No perichondrium surrounds Broyles ligament, which is connected superiorly with the thyroepiglottic ligament via fibrous extensions.[10] Inferiorly, the anterior commissure is connected to the cricothyroid ligament, a central condensation of the conus elasticus. The dense condensation of fibers that exists in this region forms a barrier to the spread of early glottic lesions, preventing erosion and further superior and inferior extension, as well as extension into the thyroid cartilage.[11] However, in more extensive lesions, the lack of perichondrium in this region, and fibrous connections superior to the thyroepiglottic ligament and inferior to the cricothyroid ligament, allow for these lesions to spread with little resistance.[3,11] Nevertheless, expanded studies based on the experience gained with transoral approaches suggest that local failures at the anterior commissure have resulted from inadequate surgical exposure and insufficient resection, rather than presumed more aggressive biologic features or deficient barriers at that level. These anatomic considerations are reflected in studies that show increased rates of local failure and recurrence in glottic lesions with anterior commissure involvement.[12,13]

Anatomic Point #2

Clinical or radiographic evidence of anterior commissure involvement should prompt the clinician to appropriate patient counseling when discussing surgical versus nonsurgical options in the management of T1, T2, and select T3 lesions.

VERTICAL PARTIAL LARYNGECTOMY

Vertical partial laryngectomies (VPLs) involve a vertical median or paramedian incision through the thyroid cartilage to gain access to the larynx at the glottic level. VPL typically involves resection of 1 or 2 vocal folds, and anterior commissure, with or without partial resection of thyroid cartilage. However, advances in access to the glottis via transoral approaches have resulted in VPL becoming predominantly of historical interest.

Indications include[14]:

1. Large T1 glottic cancers confined to a single cord
2. Small T2 glottic cancer with minimal extension into the supraglottis or subglottis
3. Early glottic lesion precluded from transoral resection due to inadequate exposure
4. Salvage surgery for early glottic recurrence in the setting of failed radiotherapy

Contraindications include[14]:

1. Involvement of the cricoarytenoid joint
2. Thyroid cartilage involvement
3. Extension of the glottic tumor to more than one-third of the contralateral cord
4. Subglottic extension greater than 5 mm

The surgical technique is as follows

1. A transverse skin incision is made
2. Subplatysmal flaps are raised in an inferior and superior direction exposing thyroid cartilage
3. A paramedian or median laryngofissure is made in thyroid cartilage
4. An excision is performed in an anterior–posterior direction to include anterior commissure, ipsilateral vocal fold up to the vocal process, and partial contralateral vocal fold (up to anterior one-third)
5. Superior–inferior extension from the vestibular fold to 5 mm below the vocal fold

Anatomic Basis

VPL surgery is predominantly utilized in resection of early glottic level lesions, with minimal subglottic/supraglottic extension, and no extension into the paraglottic space. Presently, VPL is used in the setting of inadequate visualization via transoral techniques. Paramount to appropriate oncologic margins is absence of extension beyond 5 mm into the subglottis (resection does not extend this far) and absence of vocal fold mobility impairment (indicating paraglottic space extension with thyroarytenoid muscle involvement). Furthermore, failure rates are increased in the setting of anterior commissure involvement due to the increased likelihood of subglottic and thyroid cartilage extension. Intermediate to larger-sized T2 lesions have been reported to have a failure rate of 17% to 40%, with some authors favoring supracricoid resection over VPL.[15]

HORIZONTAL PARTIAL LARYNGECTOMY

Horizontal partial laryngectomies (HPLs) involve a horizontal incision through or above the thyroid cartilage to gain access to the endolarynx. HPL is classically used for resection of glottic, transglottic, and supraglottic level carcinomas. Principally, there are 3 main variants of horizontal partial laryngectomies, in increasing order of invasiveness: (1) supraglottic partial laryngectomy, (2) supracricoid laryngectomy with cricohyoidoepiglottopexy (SCPL-CHEP), and (3) supracricoid laryngectomy with cricohyoidopexy (SCPL-CHP) (Video 2).

SUPRAGLOTTIC PARTIAL LARYNGECTOMY

Supraglottic partial laryngectomy involves resection of the pre-epiglottic space, the epiglottis, the vestibular folds, and the upper portion of the thyroid cartilage (**Fig. 2**). Reconstruction is achieved via a thyrohyoidopexy (Video 3).

Indications include

1. Early stage T1 and T2 supraglottic lesions not amenable to transoral resection due to inadequate visualization
2. Intermediate-to-large T2 lesions, with extensive contralateral extension
3. Lesions with significant supraglottic extension with possible involvement of the preepiglottic space

Contraindications include

1. Involvement of either the cricoid or thyroid cartilage
2. Fixed vocal folds
3. Impaired tongue mobility
4. Bilateral arytenoid involvement

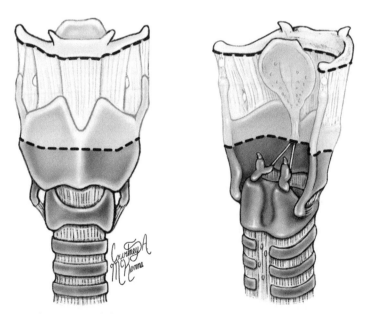

Fig. 2. Supraglottic partial laryngectomy. Involves resection of pre-epiglottic space, epiglottis, vestibular folds, and upper portion of thyroid cartilage. (Printed with permission from © Mount Sinai Health System.)

The surgical technique could be described at a glance as follows:

1. A transverse skin incision is made
2. Subplatysmal flaps are raised in an inferior and superior direction exposing the upper portion of the thyroid cartilage
3. Tracheotomy
4. A subperichondrial flap elevation is performed from the superior border of thyroid in an inferior direction
5. The inferior constrictor musculature is transected from its posterior–superior attachment to the thyroid cartilage
6. The thyroid cartilage is divided along obliquely toward the superior cornu
7. If significant pre-epiglottic space involvement is noted, the hyoid bone is included as a part of the resection margin
8. The contralateral aryepiglottic fold is transected anterior to the arytenoid cartilage
9. An incision is brought in continuity with the thyroid cartilage incision to complete resection
10. Primary reconstruction by impaction of thyroid cartilage remnant inferiorly and onto hyoid bone (thyrohyoidopexy) or tongue base superiorly

Anatomic Basis

In evaluation for candidacy of patients with supraglottic cancer for a supraglottic partial laryngectomy, accurate inferior and superior tumor mapping should be performed. Impairment of vocal fold mobility may be a clinical indication of inferior extension via the paraglottic space to involve the thyroarytenoid muscle within the glottis.[16] Supraglottic laryngectomy will not address this inferior extension and precludes this type of intervention. Studies have further verified this with increased rates of treatment failure in patients with impaired vocal cord mobility.[16] Supraglottic cancer may extend to the glottic level in 20% to 54% of cases, and thus the clinician should maintain a high index of suspicion when evaluating such patients.[16]

In order to understand superior supraglottic extension, the clinician should understand the boundaries of the pre-epiglottic space and their contribution to tumor spread. The pre-epiglottic space is bounded by the vallecula and hyoid superiorly, thyrohyoid membrane and thyroid cartilage anteriorly, the epiglottis posteriorly, and the superior aspect of the paraglottic spaces posterolaterally. Contained within the pre-epiglottic space are lymphatic and blood vessels.[17] Superior extension into the pre-epiglottic space may result in involvement of the arytenoid, aryepiglottic fold, ventricle, base of tongue, and the superior–medial aspect of the piriform sinus. Involvement of these areas may require modifications to the standard supraglottic laryngectomy technique, including partial or full resection of the hyoid bone. Furthermore, fixed or immobile tongue may indicate extension through the pre-epiglottic space to involve the tongue base muscles. In such circumstances, partial laryngectomy would be precluded due to inadequate superior margins.

Anatomic Point #3

The pre-epiglottic space may enable superior extension of cancer to involve other sites that should prompt the clinician to evaluate for possible modifications of the standard supraglottic laryngectomy.

SUPRACRICOID PARTIAL LARYNGECTOMY WITH CRICOHYOIDOEPIGLOTTOPEXY

The supracricoid partial laryngectomy (SCPL) procedure encompasses en bloc resection of bilateral paraglottic spaces (including the thyroarytenoid musculature), bilateral vocal folds, bilateral vestibular folds, the thyroid cartilage, and at most 1 arytenoid.[18] Superior extension of the resection includes the infrahyoid epiglottis and a portion of the pre-epiglottic space (**Fig. 3**). However, the suprahyoid third of the epiglottis may be spared, allowing it to be used for reconstruction via CHEP (Video 4).

Indications include[19,20]

1. Early stage T1-T2 glottic, supraglottic, or transglottic cancers not amenable to transoral resection due to inadequate exposure
2. Select T3 glottic, supraglottic, or transglottic cancers
3. Select T4 lesions with thyroid cartilage involvement of the ala, sparing the outer perichondrium

Contraindications include[15,20]

1. Extensive involvement of posterior commissure
2. Bilateral arytenoid fixation or extensive mucosal disease
3. Extralaryngeal spread
4. Invasion of hyoid bone
5. Extensive invasion of the pre-epiglottic space to include the epiglottis
6. Subglottic extension greater than 10 mm anteriorly, 5 mm laterally, or 2 mm posteriorly

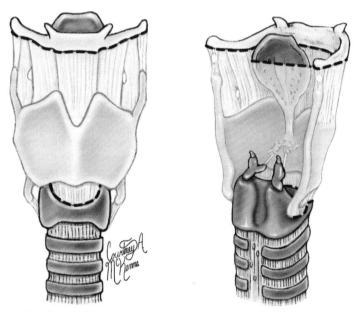

Fig. 3. Supracricoid partial laryngectomy with cricohyoidoepiglottopexy. Involves resection of bilateral paraglottic spaces, bilateral vocal folds and vestibular folds, and the thyroid cartilage. Superior extension of the resection includes the infrahyoid epiglottis and a portion of the pre-epiglottic space. (Printed with permission from © Mount Sinai Health System.)

7. Massive pre-epiglottic space involvement into the vallecula; lateral pharyngeal wall extension

The surgical technique could be described at a glance as follows:

1. A transverse skin incision is made
2. Subplatysmal flaps are raised in an inferior and superior direction exposing the thyroid cartilage
3. The trachea is mobilized and released from surrounding tissue to allow for upward mobility
4. Tracheotomy
5. The thyroid cartilage is released from all lateral attachments
6. The cricothyroid joint is disarticulated
7. Inferiorly, access to the endolarynx is achieved through the cricothyroid membrane
8. The thyrohyoid membrane is incised just above the thyroid cartilage (transepiglottic laryngotomy) to complete the resection
9. Reconstruction by impaction of cricoid cartilage inferiorly onto hyoid bone and suprahyoid epiglottis remnant superiorly (cricohyoidoepiglottopexy)

Utilization of SCPL should be considered in bulky glottic and supraglottic tumors with suspicion of extension into the paraglottic space. Furthermore, lesions with impaired or fixed vocal cord mobility should be considered for these type of procedures, as this may be an anatomic indication of glottic and paraglottic involvement. SCPL will include resection of the thyroarytenoid muscles along with the resection of bilateral paraglottic spaces. Local recurrence rates following supracricoid partial laryngectomies for T1, T2, and T3 lesions have been cited as 0%, 4.5%, and 10% respectively.[21–23]

Tucker and Smith first defined the paraglottic space as being bounded by the conus elasticus inferiorly and medially, the quadrangular membrane superiorly and medially, the thyroid cartilage anterolaterally, and the piriform sinus posteriorly.[24] The paraglottic space is a compartment that traverses the supraglottis, glottis, and subglottis, containing the ventricular saccule and the thyroarytenoid musculature. This space provides a relatively low-impedance pathway for the direct extension of laryngeal cancer.[16] Impaired vocal fold mobility may be a clinical indication of involvement of this space due to thyroarytenoid muscle involvement.[25] As tumor bulk may be a mere mechanical factor affecting vocal fold mobility, arytenoid mobility impairment should be distinctly evaluated, recognized as a more ominous finding and prompt the consideration of arytenoid resection on the involved side. However, impairment of bilateral arytenoid cartilages or massive posterior commissure involvement precludes this type of resection due to loss of both functional laryngeal units.

The intimate association of the paraglottic space with the subglottis and supraglottis may enable tumor spread and predispose to local failure. Supraglottic extension may further predispose to pre-epiglottic space involvement and thyroid cartilage invasion, contributing to treatment failure.[26–28]

Anatomic Point #4

Impaired vocal fold and arytenoid mobility may be an indication of thyroarytenoid muscle involvement and presence of tumor within the paraglottic space. The clinician should be astute to this finding, and take further care in evaluation of the supraglottis and subglottis during tumor mapping and surgical planning.

Paramount to the success and utilization of SCPL-CHEP is the absence of invasion of the pre-epiglottic space to include the epiglottis. Epiglottic involvement would prohibit the use of the epiglottis during the cricohyoidoepiglottopexy, and as such would be more amenable to SCPL-CHP.

SUPRACRICOID PARTIAL LARYNGECTOMY WITH CRICOHYOIDOPEXY

The SCPL-CHP procedure represents an extension of SCPL-CHEP resection, with added resection of the entire epiglottis and pre-epiglottic space tissue (**Fig. 4**). Reconstruction is performed by cricohyoidopexy (Video 5).

Indications include[19,20]

1. Early stage T1-T2 glottic, supraglottic, or transglottic cancers not amenable to transoral resection due to inadequate exposure
2. Select T3 glottic, supraglottic, or transglottic cancers
3. Select T4 lesions with thyroid cartilage ala involvement, sparing outer perichondrium

Contraindications include[15,20]

1. Extensive involvement of posterior commissure
2. Bilateral arytenoid fixation or extensive mucosal disease
3. Extralaryngeal spread
4. Invasion of hyoid bone
5. Subglottic extension greater than 10 mm anteriorly, 5 mm laterally, or 2 mm posteriorly
6. Massive pre-epiglottic space involvement into the vallecula; lateral pharyngeal wall extension

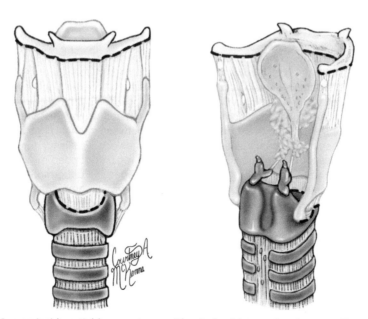

Fig. 4. Supracricoid partial laryngectomy with cricohyoidopexy. Involves resection of bilateral vocal folds and vestibular folds, the thyroid cartilage, the entire epiglottis, and pre-epiglottic tissue. (Printed with permission from © Mount Sinai Health System.)

The surgical technique could be described at a glance as follows:

1. A transverse skin incision is made
2. Subplatysmal flaps are raised in an inferior and superior direction exposing upper portion thyroid cartilage
3. The trachea is released from surrounding tissue to allow for upward mobilization
4. Tracheotomy
5. The thyroid cartilage is released from all lateral attachments
6. The cricothyroid joint is disarticulated
7. Inferiorly, access to the endolarynx is achieved through the cricothyroid membrane
8. The thyrohyoid membrane is incised just below the hyoid bone (transvallecular pharyngotomy) to complete the resection
9. Reconstruction by impaction of the cricoid cartilage inferiorly onto the hyoid bone and base of tongue superiorly (cricohyoidopexy)

Anatomic Basis

Transglottic tumors are defined as tumors traversing the ventricle, involving the vocal and vestibular folds. Transglottic lesions have an increased local failure rate of 23%.[29] This is likely because of the difficulty in determining the origin of the tumor as a true glottic lesion, or as a supraglottic lesion. True transglottic lesions should be further considered for management by supracricoid laryngectomy.

Anatomic Point #5

Transglottic tumors have an intimate association with the subglottis, supraglottis, and pre-epiglottic space. Difficulty in determining true tumor epicenter should prompt the clinician to consider supracricoid partial laryngectomy as a treatment option for these lesions.

Assessment of the subglottic space should also be assessed in lesions being considered for open conservation approaches. Strome and colleagues[30] postulated a model for the spread of lesions with significant subglottic extension based on the susceptibility of the fibroelastic barriers within the subglottis. Examination of the chondroid tissue revealed little carcinomatous involvement and minimal erosive changes. Tumors were instead found to extend through gaps between tracheal rings, respecting the boundaries of the cartilaginous tracheal framework. Similarly, tumors were enabled to spread into the paraglottic space, in the region bounded medially by the conus elasticus and laterally by the laryngeal cartilages.[30] Furthermore, lymphatic drainage of the anterior subglottis traverses the cricothyroid membrane to reach pretracheal and prelaryngeal nodes. Posterolaterally, lymphatic drainage occurs through the cricotracheal membrane to paratracheal nodes. The combination of potential for direct extension and rich lymphatic drainage may predispose to extralaryngeal spread.[31] Anatomic studies have further reinforced these considerations, as subglottic extension beyond 5 mm has been associated with higher local failure rates and cricoid cartilage involvement.[32,33]

Extensive anterior subglottic involvement may indicate extralaryngeal spread, precluding SCPL-CHP/CHEP as surgical options. Sparano and colleagues[34] determined that 100% (7 of 7) of cases with thyroid gland involvement had subglottic extension beyond 15 mm. Brennan and colleagues[2] further found that 8% (2 of 26) of tumors with greater than 5 mm subglottic extension had extralaryngeal spread to the thyroid.

Furthermore, extensive posterior subglottic extension may result in cricoid cartilage invasion, further precluding SCPL-CHP.[21] The most common site of cricoid cartilage invasion is posterior and superior, and consequently a smaller degree of subglottic extension is tolerated in this region.[35]

Anatomic Point #6

Appropriate evaluation and mapping of anterior and posterior subglottic extension should be performed to determine candidacy for SCPL-CHP. Because of the intimate relationship of the cricoid cartilage with the posterior subglottis, a smaller degree of extension in this region is tolerated.

SUMMARY

In order to appropriately manage and counsel patients with laryngeal cancer, the physician must not only be aware of the armamentarium of treatment options, but also have a thorough understanding of the complex laryngeal anatomy that impacts tumor growth and behavior. Surgical and nonsurgical approaches should be considered, with appropriate referrals made as needed. Surgical options include transoral as well as transcervical approaches. The fibroelastic framework of the larynx provides distinctive barriers that may limit tumor extension in the early stages, but guide predictable migration patterns in advanced cases. The spaces and ligaments of the larynx allow for an intricate and dynamic relationship between the subglottic, glottic, and supraglottic levels of the larynx. The paraglottic spaces form a conduit for extension to different laryngeal regions that must be understood to better determine optimal treatment options. Understanding of the distinctive anatomic associations within the larynx will enhance tumor mapping, and allow for superior outcomes.

SUPPLEMENTARY DATA

Supplementary data related to this article can be found online at http://dx.doi.org/10.1016/j.otc.2015.04.014.

REFERENCES

1. Puxeddo R, Piazza C, Mensi MC, et al. Carbon dioxide laser salvage surgery after radiotherapy failure in T1 and T2 glottic carcinoma. Otolaryngol Head Neck Surg 2004;130:84–8.
2. Brennan AJ, Meyers AD, Jafek BW. The intraoperative management of the thyroid gland during laryngectomy. Laryngoscope 1991;101:929–34.
3. Lam KH. Extralaryngeal spread of cancer of the larynx: a study with whole-organ sections. Head Neck Surg 1983;5:410–24.
4. Yeager VL, Archer CR. Anatomical routes for cacner invasion of laryngeal cartilages. Laryngoscope 1982;92(4):449–52.
5. Nakayama M. Clinical underestmation of laryngeal cancer. Arch Otolaryngol Head Neck Surg 1993;119:950–7.
6. Harrison DF. Significance and means by which laryngeal cancer invades thyroid cartilage. Ann Otol Rhinol Laryngol 1984;93:293–6.
7. Olszeweksi E. Vascularization of ossified cartilage and the spread of cancer in the larynx. Arch Otolaryngol 1976;102:200–3.

8. Piquet JJ, Chevalier D. Subtotal laryngectomy with crico-hyoido-epiglotto-pexy for the treatment of extended glottic carcinomas. Am J Surg 1991;162:357–61.
9. Kallmes D, Phillips D. The normal anterior commissure of the glottis. AJR Am J Roentgenol 1997;168:11317–9.
10. Broyles EN. The anterior commissure tendon of the larynx. Its significance in the laryngofissure operation. Preliminary note. Bull Johns Hopkins Hospital 1942;70:90.
11. Kirchner JA. Intralaryngeal barriers to the spread of cancer. Acta Otolaryngol 1987;103:503–13.
12. Laccourreye O, Weinstein G, Brasnu D. Vertical partial laryngectomy: a critical analysis of local recurrence. Ann Otol Rhinol Laryngol 1991;100:68–71.
13. Kirchner JA, Som ML. The anterior commissure technique of partial laryngectomy: clinical and laboratory observations. Laryngoscope 1975;85:1308–17.
14. Chawla S, Carney A. Organ preservation surgery for laryngeal cancer. Head Neck Oncol 2009;1:12.
15. Laccourreye O, Laccourreye L, Garcia D, et al. Vertical partial laryngectomy versus supracricoid partial laryngectomy for selected carcinomas of the true vocal cord classified as T2N0. Ann Otol Rhinol Laryngol 2000;109:965–71.
16. Weinstein G, Laccourreye O, Brasnu D. Reconsidering a paradigm: the spread of supraglottic carcinoma to the glottis. Laryngoscope 1995;105:1129–33.
17. Dayal VS, Bahri H, Stone PC. The preepiglottic space. An anatomic study. Arch Otolaryngol 1972;95:130–3.
18. Chevalier D, Piquet JJ. Subtotal laryngectomy with cricohyoidopexy for supra-glottic carcinoma: review of 61 cases. Am J Surg 1994;168:472–3.
19. Yeager LB, Grillone GA. Organ preservation surgery for intermediate size (T2 and T3) laryngeal cancer. Otolaryngol Clin North Am 2005;38:11–20.
20. Tufano RP. Organ preservation surgery for laryngeal cancer. Otolaryngol Clin North Am 2002;35:1067–80.
21. Laccourreye H, Laccourreye O, Weinstein G. Supracricoid laryngectomy with cri-cohyoidoepiglottopexy: a partial laryngeal procedure for glottic carcinoma. Ann Otol Rhinol Laryngol 1990;99:421–6.
22. Laccourreye O, Salzer SJ, Brasnu D. A clinical trial of continuous cisplatin-fluorouracil induction chemotherapy and supracricoid partial laryngectomy for glottic carcinoma. Cancer 1994;74:2781–90.
23. Laccourreye O, Salzer SJ, Brasnu D. Glottic carcinoma with a fixed true vocal cord: outcomes after neoadjuvant chemotherapy and supracricoid partial laryn-gectomy with cricohyoidoepiglottopexy. Otolaryngol Head Neck Surg 1996;114:400–6.
24. Tucker GJ, Smith HR. A histological demonstration of the development of laryn-geal connective tissue compartments. Trans Am Acad Ophthalmol Otolaryngol 1962;66:308–18.
25. Kirchner JA, Som ML. Clinical significance of fixed vocal cord. Laryngoscope 1971;81(7):1029–44.
26. Kirchner JA. One hundred laryngeal cancers studied by serial section. Laryngo-scope 1969;78:689–709.
27. Bridger GP, Nassar VH. Cancer spread in the larynx. Arch Otolaryngol 1972;95:497–505.
28. Kirchner JA. Two hundred laryngeal cacners: patterns of growht and spread as seen in serial section. Laryngoscope 1977;87:474–82.
29. Mittal B, Marks JE, Ogura J. Transglottic carcinoma. Cancer 1984;53(1):151–61.

30. Strome S, Robey T, Devancy K, et al. Subglottic carcinoma: review of a series and characerization of its patterns of spread. Ear Nose Throat J 1999;78:622–32.
31. Harrison DF. The pathology and management of subglottic cancer. Ann Otol Rhinol Laryngol 1971;80:6–12.
32. Mohr RM, Quenelle J, Shumrick DA. Vertico-frontolateral laryngectomy (hemilaryngectomy). Arch Otolaryngol Head Neck Surg 1983;109(6):384–95.
33. Glanz HK. Carcinoma of the larynx. Growth, p-classification and grading of squamous cell carcinoma of the vocal cords. Adv Otorhinolaryngol 1984;32:1–123.
34. Sparano A, Chernock R, Laccourreye O, et al. Predictors of thyroid gland invasion in glottic squamous cell carcinoma. Laryngoscope 2005;115:1247–50.
35. Welsh LW, Welsh LJ, Rizzo TA. Laryngeal spaces and lymphatics: current anatomic concepts. Ann Otol Rhinol Laryngol 1983;105:19–31.

Index

Note: Page numbers of article titles are in **boldface** type.

Otolaryngol Clin N Am 48 (2015) 717–723
http://dx.doi.org/10.1016/S0030-6665(15)00105-X
0030-6665/15/$ – see front matter © 2015 Elsevier Inc. All rights reserved.

oto.theclinics.com

M

N

Printed and bound by CPI Group (UK) Ltd, Croydon, CR0 4YY

03/10/2024

01040486-0003